ADVERSE CUTANEOUS REACTIONS TO MEDICATION

Sanford M. Goldstein, MD
Associate Clinical Professor
Department of Dermatology
University of California, San Francisco

Physician
The Kaiser Permanente Medical Group
San Francisco, California

Bruce U. Wintroub, MD
Executive Vice Dean
Professor of Dermatology
School of Medicine
University of California, San Francisco

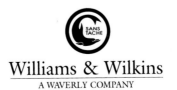

Williams & Wilkins
A WAVERLY COMPANY

BALTIMORE • PHILADELPHIA • LONDON • PARIS • BANGKOK
BUENOS AIRES • HONG KONG • MUNICH • SYDNEY • TOKYO • WROCLAW

Editor: Jonathan W. Pine, Jr.
Managing Editor: Molly L. Mullen
Typesetter: Peirce Graphic Services, Inc., Stuart, FL
Printer: Friesens, Canada

Copyright © 1996 Williams & Wilkins

351 West Camden Street
Baltimore, Maryland 21201-2436   USA

Rose Tree Corporate Center
1400 North Providence Road
Building II, Suite 5025
Media, Pennsylvania 19063-2043   USA

Printed in Canada

Library of Congress Cataloging in Publication Data

Goldstein, Sanford M. 1952–
   Adverse cutaneous reactions to medication / Sanford M. Goldstein, Bruce U.
    Wintroub.
    p. cm.
   Includes bibliographical references.
   ISBN 0-683-18042-8 (alk. paper)
   1. Dermatotoxicology. 2. Skin—Effect of drugs on. I. Wintroub, Bruce U. II. Title.
   [DNLM: 1. Drug Eruptions. 2. Drug Therapy—adverse effects. WR 165 G624a
    1996]
   RL803.G65 1996
   615'.7—dc20
   DNLM/DLC
   for Library of Congress
                                            96-4660
                                              CIP

   96 97 98 99 00
   1 2 3 4 5 6 7 8 9 10

Contents

INTRODUCTION   5

MAKING A DIAGNOSIS   6

TYPES OF ERUPTIONS   7

EXANTHEMS   7
URTICARIA   15
PHOTOSENSITIVITY   19
FIXED DRUG ERUPTION   25
LICHENOID (LICHEN PLANUS-LIKE) DRUG ERUPTION   29
PITYRIASIS ROSEA-LIKE ERUPTION   33
TOXIC EPIDERMAL NECROLYSIS (TEN)   35
ERYTHEMA MULTIFORME (EM) MAJOR
(STEVENS-JOHNSON SYNDROME)   39
EXFOLIATIVE ERYTHRODERMA   45
HYPERSENSITIVITY VASCULITIS   48
ERYTHEMA NODOSUM   52
ACNEIFORM ERUPTION   55

OTHER REACTIONS   58

HYPERTRICHOSIS/HIRSUTISM   58
DRUG-INDUCED ALOPECIA   61
HYPERPIGMENTATION   65
HYPOPIGMENTATION   70

SPECIAL SITUATIONS 72

CHEMOTHERAPY-ASSOCIATED PALMAR-PLANTAR
ERYTHRODYSESTHESIA SYNDROME (ACRAL ERYTHEMA)   72

NEUTROPHILIC ECCRINE HIDRADENITIS   73

VITAMIN K HYPERSENSITIVITY   75

ALLOPURINOL TOXICITY (HYPERSENSITIVITY) SYNDROME   77

LUPUS ERYTHEMATOSUS-LIKE REACTIONS   78

COUMARIN NECROSIS   82

ACUTE GENERALIZED EXANTHEMATOUS PUSTULOSIS   83

THE CUTANEOUS ERUPTION OF LYMPHOCYTE RECOVERY   85

ADVERSE REACTIONS AT SITES OF DRUG INJECTIONS   87

DRUGS OF PARTICULAR INTEREST 90

PENICILLINS   90

NONSTEROIDAL ANTIINFLAMMATORY DRUGS   92

MEDICATIONS USED TO TREAT HIV-RELATED DISEASES   93

CANCER CHEMOTHERAPEUTIC AGENTS   96

FUTURE DIRECTIONS 102

REPORTING ADVERSE REACTIONS 105

REFERENCES 106

ACKNOWLEDGMENTS 110

INDIVIDUAL DRUGS AND REPORTED
ADVERSE CUTANEOUS REACTIONS 111

INTRODUCTION   111

LISTING OF ADVERSE CUTANEOUS REACTIONS BY DRUG   114

INTRODUCTION

Drugs are a common exogenous cause of skin disease. Currently there is no fully satisfactory way to classify adverse cutaneous drug reactions because we do not understand the mechanisms that cause most of these reactions. The majority of drug eruptions are not caused by the classic immune mechanisms (e.g., Type I, immediate hypersensitivity; Type II, cytotoxic antibody; Type III, antigen antibody complexes; Type IV, delayed cell-mediated immunity).

METHODOLOGY

This handbook utilized extensively referenced secondary sources and reviews, as noted, as well as primary sources. Clinicians should be aware that not all side effects reported in the literature, or listed in this or other books, may actually be caused by drugs. For example, they may represent the coincidental administration of a drug with a viral or bacterial infection or another condition that itself may trigger the cutaneous reaction or with a relatively common disease such as alopecia areata, psoriasis, or atopic dermatitis. In addition, clinical-pathologic correlation may be incomplete in many reports. Many reactions are observed and reported by non-dermatologists who do not provide detailed morphologic descriptions. Finally, the rates of adverse reactions are not always compared with those of placebo. In many series, the rates of infrequent reactions, such as eczematous dermatitis, have actually been higher in the group treated with placebo, making it difficult, on the basis of these series alone, to actually attribute the reaction to the medication. It is possible that such reactions may be attributable to the underlying disease for which the drug was originally given.

DEFINITION AND APPROACH

Adverse cutaneous reactions to drugs include side effects in the skin, hair, nails, and mucous membranes that are caused by medication. While many reactions appear to be "allergic" in nature, they can range from metabolic effects (acne from anabolic steroids) to ecologic disturbance (cutaneous candidiasis after antibiotic usage). In this handbook, we classify drug eruptions according to their appearance (i.e., morphology) and review several classic morphologic reactions, essentially breaking down the topic of drug eruptions into many separate diseases, as have many previous authors. We will also discuss other selected adverse cutaneous reactions and several classes of drugs. This handbook is meant to provide an overview and to be used as a convenient clinical resource. The references listed on pp. 106–109 offer more comprehensive citations and are highly recommended and very important for the management of individual patients. Several of these, in particular Bork K, 1988, Bruinsma W, 1990, Litt JZ and Pawlak WA, Jr., 1992, and Zürcher K and Krebs A, 1992, offer clinicians ready access to several thousand journal articles covering many specific reactions. These primary sources provide essential details of clinical presentation, clinical variations, laboratory findings, and response to therapy.

GENERAL CHARACTERISTICS OF DRUG ERUPTIONS

1) They are inflammatory, and therefore generally characterized by redness or other color change.
2) They are usually widespread and symmetric.
3) When localized, they often affect specific areas, such as lower extremities, palms and soles, lips, or genital areas.

MAKING A DIAGNOSIS

1) First, consider an adverse cutaneous reaction to drugs in the differential diagnosis.

   Although a drug reaction might always be included in the differential diagnosis, it should be carefully considered in four specific situations:

   a. When use of a medication is closely followed by one of the classic morphologic patterns associated with drug eruptions (e.g., urticaria, morbilliform, photosensitivity, etc.).

   b. When a typical, usually rare, skin disease presents in a patient taking a medication known to cause that disease (e.g., pemphigus and penicillamine).

   c. When a patient presents with an atypical, widespread skin disease that is not readily classifiable as a particular classic dermatologic entity (e.g., psoriasis-like rash in a patient taking a beta blocker).

   d. When a preexistent skin disease worsens in a patient taking a drug known to cause such exacerbations (e.g., lithium and psoriasis; iodine and dermatitis herpetiformis; certain oral contraceptives and acne).

2) Describe and classify the morphology of the eruption.

3) Rule out other causes of the rash—e.g., does the HIV-infected patient with an itchy, bumpy rash on trimethoprim-sulfamethoxazole have scabies or a folliculitis?

4) List all drugs that the patient is taking or has taken recently—include all suppositories, eye and nose drops, topicals, and OTC drugs.

5) Determine the temporal relationship between drug administration and onset of the eruption (the duration between administration and appearance of the reaction will vary with each reaction).

6) Determine the likelihood of each drug causing that particular eruption based on controlled studies and case reports.

7) Follow the response to stopping the medication. The time required for clearing of the reaction may vary with each type of reaction.

EXANTHEMS

(MACULOPAPULAR, MORBILLIFORM ERUPTIONS)

DESCRIPTION

Flat and/or barely raised red spots of one to several mm. In some cases the spots may be 1 cm or larger. May or may not be pruritic.

May present as confluent red areas, or become confluent in areas, with time. Should be bilateral and symmetric.

Often begin on the head/neck or upper torso and proceed down the body.

Often have a sudden onset in the first two weeks of administration, except for semisynthetic penicillins, which may have their onset after the first 2 weeks of administration.

Represent the most common type of cutaneous drug eruption.

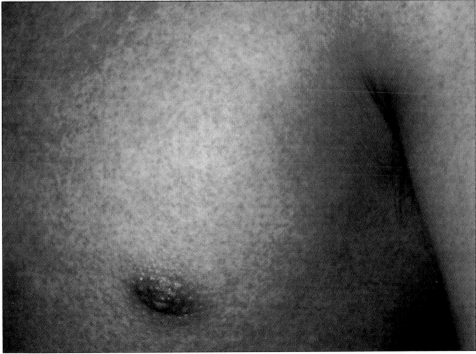

Figure 1. Exanthem due to penicillin.

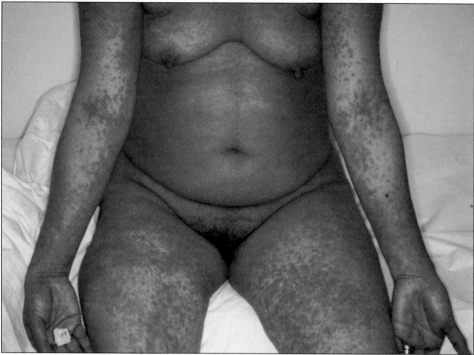

Figure 2. Exanthem due to sulfas in a patient sensitized by AVC (sulfanilamide) cream.

DIFFERENTIAL DIAGNOSIS

Viral exanthem is the most common differential diagnosis.

Secondary syphilis (uncommon). Check palms/soles, mucous membranes for lesions typical of syphilis.

Eruption due to lymphocyte recovery after chemotherapy of leukemia.

MECHANISM

Unknown. There is little evidence that this type of reaction represents true allergy, although recent studies suggest that some patients may have positive patch tests (presumably Type IV hypersensitivity) to diluted drug.

A high incidence of drug-induced exanthems occurs:

>   With ampicillin administration in patients with infectious mononucleosis.

>   With trimethoprim-sulfamethoxazole administration in patients with HIV infection.

LABS

Not useful.

MANAGEMENT

Stop all medications that are not required and stop the drug(s) most likely to cause the eruption.

Substitute unrelated medications.

In cases in which no good substitute is available, consider continuing treatment with careful follow-up. (This most commonly applies to multiply infected, critically ill patients taking multiple drugs, such as bone marrow transplant patients.)

PROGNOSIS

Resolution in 7 to 14 days. Very rare progression to a more serious reaction (e.g., erythroderma).

The following tables are best used to compare the relative rates at which different drugs cause exanthems or urticaria and do not indicate the absolute ability of a drug to cause a reaction. For example, aspirin caused no reactions in 984 recipients (see Table 6), but is a well-known cause of urticaria.

TABLE 1. ALLERGIC SKIN REACTIONS TO DRUGS RECEIVED BY AT LEAST 1000 PATIENTS.

Drug	No. of Reactions	No. of Recipients	Reaction Rate*	95% Confidence Intervals
Amoxicillin	63	1225	51.4	39.0 -63.8
Trimethoprim-sulfamethoxazole	36	1066	33.8	23.6 -46.7
Ampicillin	59	1775	33.2	24.9 -41.5
Blood	24	1112	21.6	13.8 -32.1
Dipyrone	13	3279	4.0	2.1 - 6.7
Atropine sulfate	2 †	1231	1.6	0.2 - 5.8
Mefruside	2	1229	1.6	0.2 - 5.9
Nitrazepam	5	3441	1.5	0.46- 3.4
Furosemide	2	3830	0.5	0.06- 1.9
Diazepam	2	4707	0.4	0.05- 1.5
Potassium chloride	1 †	3460	0.3	0.01- 1.6

* Reactions per 1000 recipients.
† Urticaria, proved by rechallenge.

Drugs with the highest rates of exanthems and urticaria.
Drug reaction rates taken from the Boston Collaborative Drug Surveillance Program.
Reprinted with permission from *JAMA* (1986; 256:3358-3363), Copyright © 1986, American Medical Association, Bigby M, Jick S, Jick H, Arndt K. Reaction rates vary somewhat compared to an earlier report, Arndt KA and Jick H. *JAMA* (1976; 235:918-923).

TABLE 2. ALLERGIC SKIN REACTIONS TO DRUGS RECEIVED BY 500 TO 999 PATIENTS.

Drug	No. of Reactions	No. of Recipients	Reaction Rate*	95% Confidence Intervals
Semisynthetic penicillin	14	676	20.7	11.4 -34.8
Penicillin G	17	918	18.5	10.8 -29.6
Acetylcysteine	7	791	8.8	3.5 -18.2
Allopurinol	6	784	7.7	2.8 -16.7
Bromhexine hydrochloride	4	627	6.4	1.8 -16.3
Gentamicin sulfate	3	670	4.5	0.93-13.1
Pentazocine hydrochloride	4	885	4.5	1.2 -11.5
Barbiturates	2	505	4.0	0.5 -14.3
Metoclopramide hydrochloride	3	929	3.2	0.7 - 9.5
Heparin sodium	1	899	1.1	0.03- 6.2

* Reactions per 1000 recipients.

Drugs with the highest rates of exanthems and urticaria. Drug reaction rates taken from the Boston Collaborative Drug Surveillance Program. Reprinted with permission from *JAMA* (1986; 256:3358-3363), Copyright © 1986, American Medical Association, Bigby M, Jick S, Jick H, Arndt K.

TABLE 3. ALLERGIC SKIN REACTIONS TO DRUGS RECEIVED BY 100 TO 499 PATIENTS.

Drug	No. of Reactions	No. of Recipients	Reaction Rate*	95% Confidence Intervals
Ipodate	5	180	27.8	8.9 -65.0
Cephalosporins	10	473	21.1	10.1 -38.9
Erythromycin	3	147	20.4	4.2 -59.9
Dihydrallazine hydrochloride	3	157	19.1	3.9 -56.1
Cyanocobalamin	3	168	17.9	3.7 -52.4
Quinidine	4	298	13.4	3.7 -34.2
Hyoscine butylbromide	3	227	13.2	2.7 -38.8
Cimetidine	3	235	12.8	2.6 -37.4
Phenylbutazone	2	172	11.6	1.4 -41.9
Phenazopyridine hydrochloride	1	113	8.8	0.2 -49.6
Hydralazine hydrochloride	1	120	8.3	0.2 -46.7
Carbocysteine	2	294	6.8	0.81-24.5
Analgesic mixture†	3	445	6.7	1.4 -19.8
Vincristine sulfate	1	160	6.3	0.16-35.0
Isoniazid	1	180	5.6	0.14-31.1
Cyclophosphamide	1	210	4.8	0.12-26.7
Doxycycline	2	425	4.7	0.56-16.9
Glyburide	1	477	2.1	0.05-11.7
Indomethacin	1	482	2.1	0.05-11.6

* Reactions per 1000 recipients.
† Metamizole, ethenzamide codeine, pitofenone, and fenpipramide (Baralgin).

Drug reaction rates taken from the Boston Collaborative Drug Surveillance Program. Reprinted with permission from *JAMA* (1986; 256:3358-3363), Copyright © 1986, American Medical Association, Bigby M, Jick S, Jick H, Arndt K.

TABLE 4. ALLERGIC SKIN REACTIONS TO DRUGS RECEIVED BY FEWER THAN 100 PATIENTS.

Drug	No. of Reactions	No. of Recipients
Phenazopyridine hydrochloride-sulfisoxazole	1	10
Diatrizoate	1	4
Methimazole	1	47
Pentoxifylline	1	41
Pizotyline	1	2
Plasma (protein fraction)	1	14
Platelets	13	29
Practolol	2	74
Rifampin	1	84
Diatrizoate meglumine or sodium (Urografin)	3	9

Drug reaction rates taken from the Boston Collaborative Drug Surveillance Program. Reprinted with permission from *JAMA* (1986; 256:3358-3363), Copyright © 1986, American Medical Association, Bigby M, Jick S, Jick H, Arndt K.

TABLE 5. DRUGS RECEIVED BY MORE THAN 1000 PATIENTS WITH NO ALLERGIC SKIN REACTIONS.

Drug	No. of Recipients
Digoxin	4716
Antacid*	1794
Promethazine hydrochloride	1630
Acetaminophen	1600
Spironolactone	1291
Nitroglycerin	1254
Methyldopa	1234
Isosorbide dinitrate	1173
Meperidine hydrochloride	1157
Aminophylline	1112
Propranolol hydrochloride	1051
Prednisolone	1001

* Aluminum hydroxide, magnesium hydroxide, and simethicone (Gelusil, Maalox Plus).

Drug reaction rates taken from the Boston Collaborative Drug Surveillance Program. Reprinted with permission from *JAMA* (1986; 256:3358-3363), Copyright © 1986, American Medical Association, Bigby M, Jick S, Jick H, Arndt K.

TABLE 6. DRUGS RECEIVED BY 500 TO 999 PATIENTS WITH NO ALLERGIC SKIN REACTIONS.

Drug	No. of Recipients
Aspirin	984
Potassium iodide	879
Flurazepam hydrochloride	872
Insulin injection	835
Prednisone	690
Magnesium sulfate	631
Prochlorperazine	600
Diphenhydramine	599
Codeine	596
Docusate sodium	586
Ferrous sulfate	553
Milk of magnesia	503

Drug reaction rates taken from the Boston Collaborative Drug Surveillance Program. Reprinted with permission from *JAMA* (1986; 256:3358-3363), Copyright © 1986, American Medical Association, Bigby M, Jick S, Jick H, Arndt K.

TABLE 7. DRUGS RECEIVED BY 100 TO 499 PATIENTS WITH NO ALLERGIC SKIN REACTIONS.

Drug	No. of Recipients	Drug	No. of Recipients
Hydrocortisone	486	Guaifenesin	184
Phosphate enema	469	Diphenoxylate hydrochloride, atropine sulfate	172
Morphine sulfate	452		
Castor oil	414	Chlorpromazine	167
Multivitamins	413	Theophylline	167
Glycerin suppositories	403	Chlorothiazide	165
Bisacodyl	376	Nystatin	165
Aluminum hydroxide gel	369	Sorbitol solution	165
Warfarin sodium	336	Propoxyphene	164
Hydroxyzine	332	Chloramphenicol	162
Phytonadione	307	Amitriptyline hydrochloride	159
Ascorbic acid	288	Chlordiazepoxide	157
Vitamin B complex	276	Sulfasalazine	154
Lidocaine hydrochloride	272	Potassium perchlorate	151
Thiamine hydrochloride	265	Papaverine hydrochloride	148
Magnesium citrate	264	Oxycodone, aspirin	143
Chloral hydrate	263	Pyridoxine hydrochloride	143
Tolbutamine	251	Magaldrate	141
Tetracycline	246	Chlorpropamide	140
Reserpine	246	Mineral oil	128
Phenytoin sodium	241	Neomycin sulfate	128
Hydrochlorothiazide	226	Opium tincture	126
Thyroid	217	Procainamide hydrochloride	126
Folic acid	208	Multivitamin	117
Insulin suspension, isophane	203	Insulin zinc suspension	116
Papaveretum	202	Serum albumin, human	113
Dexamethasone	192	Nitrofurantoin	104
Polystrene sodium sulfonate	191	Thioridazine	103
Levothyroxine sodium	186	Oxtriphylline	100

Drug reaction rates taken from the Boston Collaborative Drug Surveillance Program. Reprinted with permission from *JAMA* (1986; 256:3358-3363), Copyright © 1986, American Medical Association, Bigby M, Jick S, Jick H, Arndt K.

URTICARIA

DESCRIPTION

Pruritic red wheals of 1 to many cm that may form complex patterns as they appear and resolve. Individual lesions should last 24 hours or less.

May be accompanied by angioedema of lips or eyelids.

May progress to anaphylaxis or an anaphylactoid reaction.

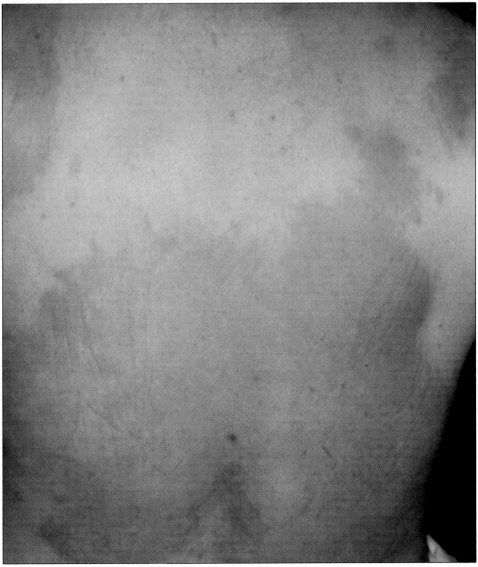

Figure 3. Large urticarial plaque.

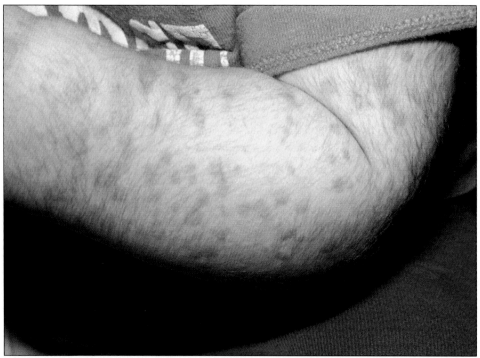

Figure 4. Urticaria caused by amoxicillin/clavulanate potassium.

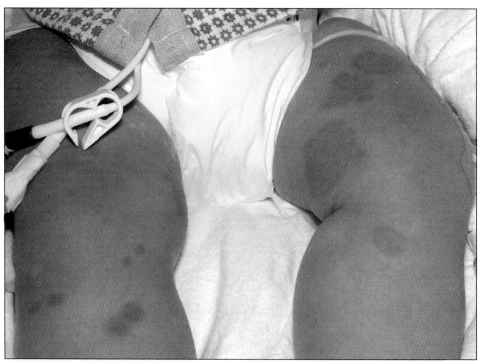

Figure 5. Urticaria during infusion of antithymosite globulin.

DIFFERENTIAL DIAGNOSIS

Idiopathic urticaria.

Urticaria due to foods, parasites, viral (hepatitis) or bacterial infections, etc.

Rare physical urticarias (due to sunlight, cold, heat, vibration, pressure, and water).

Cholinergic urticaria (due to a rise in body temperature with exercise and/or rise in skin temperature, e.g., hot shower). These often have a typical appearance: small wheals and large red flares.

Contact urticaria (caused by topical contact with foods, flavorings, latex rubber, etc.).

Urticarial vasculitis (a form of cutaneous vasculitis suspected when individual lesions last > 24 hours and have purpura within them).

Dermographism (linear hives caused by friction/scratching).

Erythema multiforme minor (acral target lesions; individual lesions last > 24 hours).

MECHANISM

IgE-mediated or direct, non-IgE-mediated activation of mast cells.

LABS

Seldom helpful. CBC/sedimentation rate is one approach to the initial workup.

MANAGEMENT

Stop the drug; do not substitute a related medication.

If rapidly progressing: epinephrine 1:1000 0.3 ml subQ. with noting of contraindications. Emergent care as needed.

Antihistamines (H_1 blockers) around the clock.

Patient education regarding medicines that may cross-react with the suspected offender. As with all adverse cutaneous reactions, particularly severe ones, update all medical records. Report the reaction to the appropriate pharmacy or hospital committee, if available. Consider use of a MedicAlert® bracelet for severe reactions.

DRUGS THAT COMMONLY CAUSE URTICARIA

Many drugs can cause urticaria

Likely offenders include:

> Antibiotics, especially penicillins
>
> Aspirin
>
> Blood products
>
> Captopril
>
> Nonsteroidal antiinflammatory drugs
>
> Cancer chemotherapeutic agents such as asparaginase and antithymocyte globulin
>
> Iodine contrast media

Some agents may activate mast cells directly via a non-IgE-mediated mechanism:

> Alcohol
>
> Aminoglycoside antibiotics
>
> Amphetamine
>
> Aspirin
>
> Atropine
>
> Curare, succinylcholine
>
> Dextrans
>
> Opiates
>
> Papaverine
>
> Polymyxin B
>
> Quinine
>
> Radiocontrast media
>
> Rifampin
>
> Thiamine
>
> Thiopental
>
> Tolazoline
>
> Vancomycin

PHOTOSENSITIVITY

DESCRIPTION

Any eruption that is prominent on the face, dorsal hands, "V" of the neck and upper chest (presternal area) should suggest an adverse reaction to light. This distribution is key to the diagnosis.

Initially the eruption spares under the chin, under the nose, and inside the fold of the upper eyelids. (The eruption may involve these areas if the rash is chronic.)

All light-exposed areas, such as the face and hands, need not be affected equally.

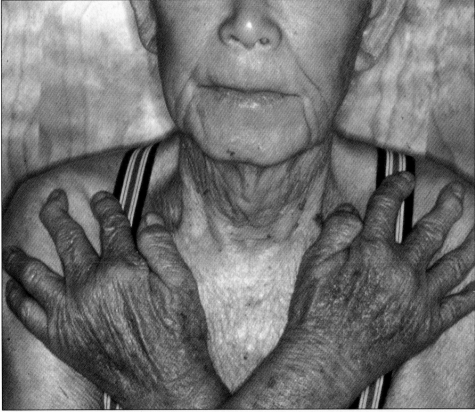

Figure 6. Photosensitivity to hydrochlorothiazide presenting as red papules and plaques on face, neck, and hands.

The eruption may have one of many appearances:

> Simulating a bad sunburn; this is a "phototoxic" reaction, the most common type of drug-induced photosensitivity, and not a form of allergy. Theoretically, it would occur in anyone, given enough drug and light.

> Consisting of small or large papules or plaques.

> Becoming vesicular, scaly or weepy.

Patients with phototoxicity reactions are commonly sensitive to ultraviolet A (UVA radiation), the so-called "tanning rays" at 320-400 nm. Patients with true photoallergy, that is, the interaction of drug, light, and the immune system, a less common form of drug-induced photosensitivity, are often sensitive to UVB, the so-called "burning rays" at 290-320 nm.

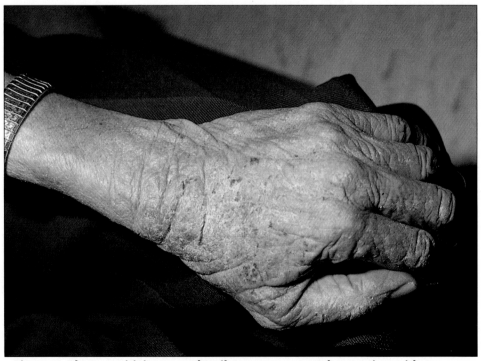

Figure 7. Photosensitivity to enalapril presents as a scaly eruption with a sharp cutoff at the wrists. The face was similarly involved.

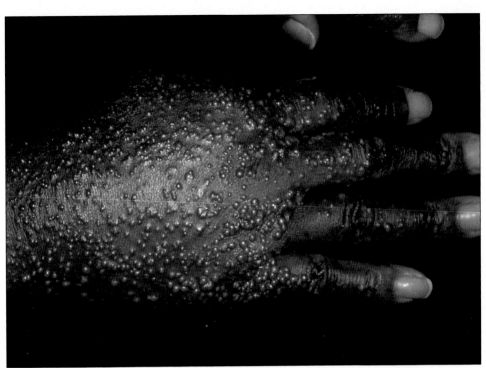

Figure 8. Photosensitivity to piroxicam presents as a vesicular eruption on the hand.

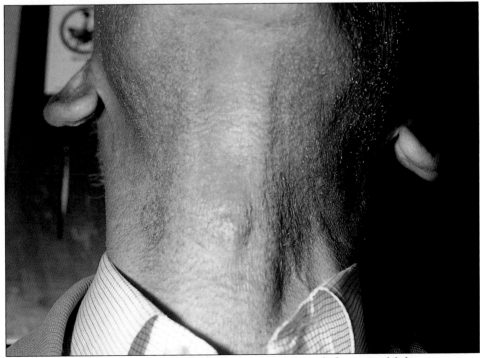

Figure 9. Sparing underneath the chin is suggestive of photosensitivity.

DIFFERENTIAL DIAGNOSIS

Polymorphous light eruption (PMLE).

Systemic lupus erythematosis (SLE).

Porphyria cutanea tarda.

Photosensitivity caused by a contact allergen (photoallergic contact dermatitis).

LABS

Skin biopsy for PMLE and SLE.

Phototesting is important to document light sensitivity and to characterize the causative wavelengths. In cases of obvious drug-induced photosensitivity, it is probably necessary only if the photosensitivity persists after discontinuation of the drug.

Photopatch testing for photocontact allergy if suspected from the history.

Serologic workup for SLE when clinically indicated.

Direct immunofluorescence test for SLE on skin biopsies may be falsely positive if performed on sun-exposed skin.

MANAGEMENT

For the patient on a new medication that is likely to cause photosensitivity, stop the drug. If there is a poor response to drug dechallenge, or if there is no obvious drug exposure, refer the patient for further evaluation as described above. Sunscreens may be helpful in patients sensitive to wavelengths in the UVB range, but they are less helpful in preventing photoeruptions due to UVA. Photosensitivity may persist for weeks or months after dechallenge.

DRUGS LIKELY TO CAUSE PHOTOSENSITIVITY

Thiazides

Sulfonamides

Furosemide

Nonsteroidal antiinflammatory drugs

Tetracyclines (except minocycline)

Phenothiazines

Other drugs that may cause photosensitivity

Amantadine
Amiodarone
Amitriptyline
Arsenic
Astemizole
Azatadine
Azathioprine
Bismuth
Bumetanide
Captopril
Carbamazepine
Carbinoxamine
Chloral hydrate
Chloramphenicol
Chlordiazepoxide
Chlorhexidine
Chloroquine
Chlorpromazine
Chlorpropamide
Chlorprothixene
Chlortetracycline
Chlorthalidone
Ciprofloxacin
Clemastine
Clindamycin
Clofazimine
Clofibrate
Codeine
Copper
Corticosteroids
Cromolyn sodium
Cyclophosphamide
Cyproheptadine
Dapsone
Decarbazine
Demeclocycline

Desipramine
Diazepam
Diazoxide
Diclofenac
Diethylstilbestrol
Diflunisal
Diphenhydramine
Disopyramide
Doxepin
Doxycycline
Enalapril
Enoxacin
Ethionamide
Etretinate
Fansidar
Fluorescein
5-Fluorouracil
Flurbiprofen
Furosemide
Gentamicin
Gold
Griseofulvin
Haloperidol
Hydralazine
Hydrochlorothiazide
Imipramine
Indomethacin
Interferon alpha (2a or 2b)
Isocarboxazid
Isoniazid (INH)
Isotretinoin
Ketoprofen
Lincomycin
Meclofenamate
Meclofenamate sodium
Meperidine

Meprobamate
Mercaptopurine
Mercury
Mesoridazine
Mestranol + Norethindrone
Methotrexate
Methoxsalen plus UV light (PUVA)
Methyldopa
Methylphenidate
Minocycline
Nalidixic acid
Naproxen
Nifedipine
Nitrofurantoin
Norfloxacin
Nortriptyline
Ofloxacin
Oral contraceptive agents
Oxytetracycline
Penicillins
Perphenazine
Phenelzine
Phenobarbital
Phenytoin (diphenylhydantoin)
Piroxicam
Procaine
Procarbazine
Prochlorperazine
Promazine
Promethazine
Propylthiouracil
Protriptyline

Pyrazinamide
Pyritinol
Quinethazone
Quinidine
Quinine
Reserpine
Silver
Simvastatin
Streptomycin
Sulfadiazine (tablets)
Sulfadoxine
Sulfanilamide
Sulfasalazine
Sulfathiazole
Sulfisoxazole
Sulindac
Thioguanine
Thioridazine
Thiothixene
Tiopronin
Tolbutamide
Triamterene
Trimethadione
Trimethoprim
Trimethoprim + Sulfamethoxazole
Tripelennamine
Triprolidine
Valproic acid
Verapamil
Vinblastine
Vitamin A

FIXED DRUG ERUPTION

DESCRIPTION

Solitary or multiple red macules or plaques that are often tender and occur in the same place each time a particular medication is administered. The plaques may be one to many cm in size. Recurrence in the same location is the key to diagnosis.

The face or the glans penis is commonly affected, but any location is possible.

Often, but not always, leaves an area of hyperpigmentation in the affected area during resolution.

Rarely blisters centrally.

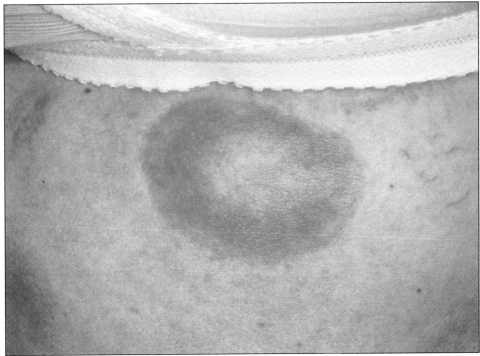

Figure 10. Fixed drug eruption from phenolphthalein. Fixed drug eruptions often hyperpigment during resolution.

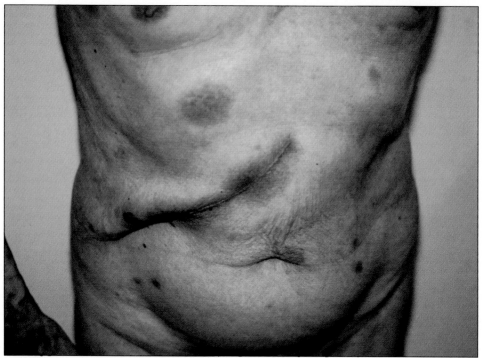

Figure 11. Fixed drug eruption with multiple lesions.

DIFFERENTIAL DIAGNOSIS

Erythema multiforme.

LABS

Skin biopsy may be diagnostic.

MANAGEMENT

Discontinue medication.
Potent topical steroids may be of benefit.

DRUGS THAT ARE COMMON CAUSES OF FIXED DRUG ERUPTION

Ampicillin
Aspirin
Barbiturates
Metronidazole
Nonsteroidal antiinflammatory drugs
Oral contraceptives
Phenolphthalein
Sulfonamides
Tetracyclines

DRUGS THAT MAY CAUSE FIXED DRUG ERUPTIONS

Acetaminophen
Allopurinol
Amphetamine
Ampicillin
Antimony
Antipyrine
Aprobarbital
Arsenic
Aspirin
Atropine
Bisacodyl
Bismuth
Bromine
Bromsulfalein
Carbamazepine
Carbinoxamine
Carisoprodol
Chloral hydrate
Chlordiazepoxide
Chlormezanone
Chloroquine
Chlorpromazine
Chlortetracycline
Codeine
Corticosteroids
Cyclizine
Dapsone
Demeclocycline
Dextran
Diazepam
Diethylstilbestrol
Digoxin
Dimenhydrinate
Diphenhydramine
Disulfiram
Doxycycline
Ephedrine
Epinephrine
Erythromycin
Estrogens
Ethchlorvynol
Ethotoin
Foscarnet
Gluthetimide
Gold
Griseofulvin
Guanethidine
Hydralazine

Hydroxyurea
Ibuprofen
Imipramine
Iodine
Ketoconazole
Magnesium
Meclofenamate
Meclofenamate sodium
Mefenamic acid
Menthol
Meprobamate
Mercury
Mesna
Methamphetamine
Methaqualone
Methenamine
Methenamine-hippurate
Methyldopa
Metronidazole
Minocycline
Naproxen
Nicotinic acid (Niacin)
Nifedipine
Nitrofurantoin
Nystatin
Oral contraceptive agents
Oxytetracycline
Paramethadione
Penicillin G
Penicillin V

Penicillins
Pentaerythritol tetranitrate
Pentobarbital
Phenobarbital
Phenytoin (diphenylhydantoin)
Piroxicam
Prednisolone
Prochlorperazine
Promethazine
Propylthiouracil
Quinacrine
Quinidine
Quinine
Reserpine
Streptomycin
Sulfadiazine (tablets)
Sulfamethoxazole
Sulfamethoxypyridazine
Sulfanilamide
Sulfathiazole
Sulfisoxazole
Sulindac
Tetracycline
Thiopental
Tolbutamide
Trimethadione
Trimethoprim
Trimethoprim + Sulfamethoxazole
Tripelennamine
Vaccine: Typhus/Paratyphus

LICHENOID (LICHEN PLANUS-LIKE) DRUG ERUPTION

DESCRIPTION

Multiple violaceous, discrete, flat-topped papules that may be polygonal in shape. Some lichenoid eruptions are less discrete, but are comprised of violaceous plaques that are larger than idiopathic lichen planus.

When used clinically, the word "lichenoid" refers to papules of this color and shape; used histologically, the word describes a "band-like" infiltrate of lymphocytes at the junction of the dermis and epidermis that is seen in clinical lichenoid or lichen planus-like eruptions.

Lesions may be generalized, photodistributed, or involve the oral mucosa.

Often pruritic.

The onset may be weeks to months to years after administration of a drug.

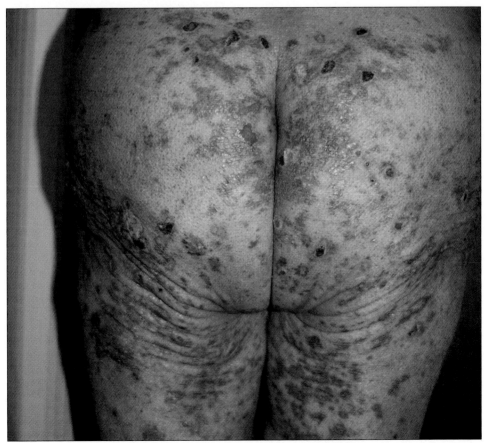

Figure 12. Lichenoid drug eruption due to chlorpropamide.

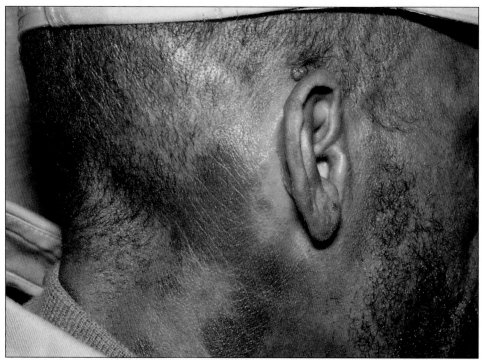

Figure 13. Photolichenoid drug eruption.

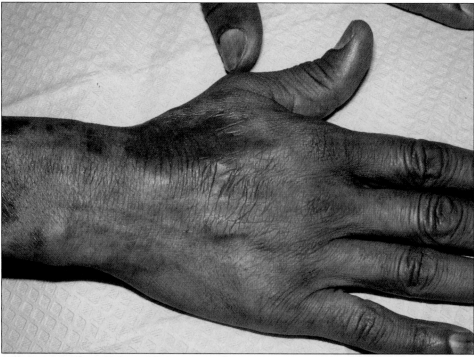

Figure 14. Photolichenoid drug eruption.

Differential diagnosis

Lichen planus.

Graft versus host disease.

Labs

Skin biopsy can determine if the histologic pattern is lichenoid, and occasionally may distinguish between lichenoid drug eruption and true lichen planus, but not when the lichenoid drug eruption is photodistributed.

Management

Discontinue medication if possible. There are rare reports of spontaneous clearing despite continuation of drug. Resolution may occur months after dechallenge.

Treat with a medium-to-high potency topical steroid.

Drugs that most commonly cause lichenoid drug eruptions

Antimalarials

Chlorpropamide

Furosemide

Gold

Methyldopa

Phenothiazines

Quinidine

Thiazides

Tolazamide

OTHER DRUGS THAT MAY CAUSE LICHENOID ERUPTIONS

Acetazolamide
Acyclovir
Arsenic
Aspirin
Bismuth
Bleomycin
Captopril (oral mucosal lichenoid reaction)
Carbamazepine
Chloral hydrate
Chlordiazepoxide
Chloroquine
Chlorpromazine
Chlorpropamide
Cinnarizine
Colchicine
Copper
Cyclophosphamide
Cyproheptadine
Dapsone
Demeclocycline
Diazoxide
Ethambutol
Fansidar
Fenbufen
5-Fluorouracil
Flurbiprofen
Furosemide
Gold
Griseofulvin
Hydrochlorothiazide
Hydroxychloroquine
Hydroxyurea
Imipramine
Indomethacin

Iodine
Isoniazid (INH)
Labetalol
Levamisole
Mercaptopurine
Mercury
Methenamine
Methyldopa
Naproxen
Oral contraceptives
Penicillamine
Penicillins
Phenytoin (diphenylhydantoin)
Pindolol
Prazosin
Propranolol
Propylthiouracil
Pyrimethamine
Pyritinol
Quinacrine
Quinidine (lichenoid photosensitive eruption)
Quinine
Spironolactone
Streptomycin
Sulindac
Tetracycline
Tiopronin
Tolazamide
Tolbutamide
Tripelennamine
Triprolidine
Vaccine: Cholera
Verapamil

PITYRIASIS ROSEA-LIKE ERUPTION

DESCRIPTION

Multiple round to oval patches with central collarette scale or "cigarette paper" wrinkled appearance, located on the trunk, and to a lesser extent, the extremities. They lack the dense, white scaling typical of psoriasis.

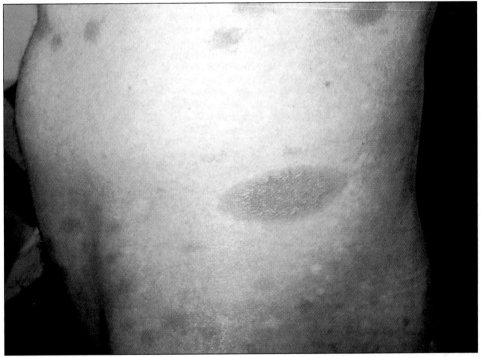

Figure 15. Pityriasis rosea.

Differential diagnosis

Pityriasis rosea.

Secondary syphilis (check palms/soles/mucosa).

Labs

Skin biopsy may be helpful. Serologies can rule out syphilis.

Management

Discontinue medication or lower the dose.

Drugs that may cause pityriasis rosea-like eruptions

Barbiturates

Bismuth compounds

Captopril

Clonidine

Gold

Griseofulvin

Isotretinoin

Labetalol

Meprobamate

Metronidazole

Penicillins

Tripelennamine

TOXIC EPIDERMAL NECROLYSIS (TEN)

DESCRIPTION

Sudden onset of large, red, tender areas.

Rapid progression to blistering and denudation.

Muscosal areas and the eyes are often affected.

The patient will demonstrate a positive Nikolsky's sign (i.e., separation of the epidermis on stroking the skin with firm pressure using a cotton applicator or other instrument).

A recently proposed consensus definition of TEN includes cases with epidermal detachment > 10% of body surface area with large epidermal sheets and no macules or target lesions and cases with widespread flat atypical targets or macules with > 30% of body surface area with epidermal detachment (Bastuji-Garin, Rzany B, Stern RS, et al 1993). See Table 8, p. 42.

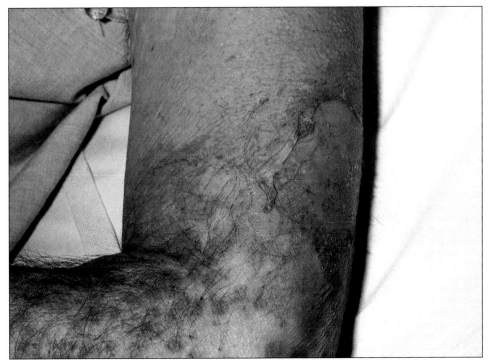

Figure 16. Toxic epidermal necrolysis. The patient demonstrates blisters and denuded skin.

Differential diagnosis

TEN associated with graft versus host disease.

Erythema multiforme major (Stevens-Johnson syndrome). (The nosologic relationship of Stevens-Johnson syndrome and TEN is an area of controversy and investigation.) See p. 39.

Staph scalded skin syndrome can readily be distinguished from TEN.

Labs

Immediate diagnosis may be made on frozen section of a skin biopsy or of a fresh blister roof, demonstrating a subepidermal blister.

Management

If denudation is widespread, optimal management includes metabolic and fluid management, avoidance of infection, and meticulous skin care, as available in a burn unit. Denuded skin may be covered by use of porcine xenografts, if necessary, but split thickness skin grafts are generally not indicated. Eye care is essential.

Systemic steroids do not appear to be efficacious, but some clinicians advocate the use of pulse corticosteroid therapy.

Some preliminary reports have suggested that cyclophosphamide plus prednisone may be the treatment of choice early in the course of TEN. Other reports suggest that plasmapheresis or intravenous pentoxifylline may also halt further progression of this reaction.

Prognosis

Mortality can be as high as 75% in the elderly, but has been quoted at approximately 25-30% overall.

Age, the percent of surface area that is denuded, and blood urea nitrogen (BUN) value are prognostic factors.

Ocular, mucosal and cutaneous sequelae are common.

Drugs that are the most common causes of TEN

Allopurinol

Ampicillin/Amoxicillin

Nonsteroidal antiinflammatory drugs

Phenobarbital

Phenytoin (diphenylhydantoin)

Sulfonamides

Other drugs reported to cause TEN

Acetazolamide
Antipyrine
Aspirin
Benzathine penicillin
Benzocaine
Captopril
Carbamazepine
Chlorambucil
Chloramphenicol
Chlormezanone
Chloroquine
Chlorpromazine
Chlorpropamide
Chlortetracycline
Chlorthalidone
Cimetidine
Ciprofloxacin
Clofibrate
Clonazepam
Codeine
Cyclophosphamide
Dactinomycin
Dapsone
Dexbrompheniramine
Diclofenac
Diflunisal
Diltiazem
Diphenhydramine
Erythromycin
Ethambutol
Fansidar
Fenbufen

Fenoprofen
5-Fluorouracil
Flurbiprofen
Gold
Griseofulvin
Hydrochlorothiazide
Hydroxychloroquine
Ibuprofen
Indomethacin
Isoniazid (INH)
L-Asparaginase
Meperidine
Mephenytoin
Meprobamate
Mercaptopurine
Methotrexate
Methyldopa
Mithramycin
Nalidixic acid
Neomycin
Nitrofurantoin
Norfloxacin
Penicillamine
Penicillins
Pentazocine
Phenolphthalein
Piroxicam
Prednisone
Primodone
Procaine
Procaine penicillin
Procarbazine

Promethazine
Propranolol
Pyrimethamine
Pyritinol
Quinidine
Quinine
Rifampin
Salicylamide
Simvastatin
Streptomycin
Streptozocin
Sulfadiazine (tablets)
Sulfadoxine
Sulfamethizole
Sulfasalazine
Sulfathiazole
Sulfisoxazole

Sulindac
Tetracycline
Thiabendazole
Thiacetazone
Tolbutamide
Tolmetin
Trimethoprim
Trimethoprim +
Sulfamethoxazole
Vaccine: BCG
Vaccine: Diphtheria antitoxin
Vaccine: Diphtheria-Pertussis-
Tetanus toxoid (DTP)
Vaccine: Measles
Vaccine: Poliomyelitis (Salk)
Vaccine: Tetanus antitoxin
Vancomycin

ERYTHEMA MULTIFORME (EM) MAJOR (STEVENS-JOHNSON SYNDROME)

DESCRIPTION

A recent study documented that clinicians have often used their own unique approaches toward diagnosing EM (or EM minor), EM major and TEN. Even among experts, the definition and recognition of a target lesion is variable. These syndromes are now being studied in a prospective manner by splitting out and categorizing lesions according to multiple features defined by an illustrated atlas (Bastuji-Garins, Rzany B, Stern RS, et al 1993).

The proposed consensus definition (*Ibid.*) of lesions found in EM includes:

1. Target lesions: "individual lesions less than 3 cm in diameter with a round regular shape, well defined border, and at least 3 different zones, i.e., two concentric rings around a central disk" (*Ibid.*). These are most often associated with post-herpetic EM minor and are not seen in TEN. See Fig. 17.

2. Raised atypical targets: "round edematous, palpable lesions reminiscent of EM, with only 2 zones and/or a poorly defined border" (*Ibid.*). See Fig. 18.

3. Flat atypical targets: as in raised atypical targets but flat or with a central blister. See Fig. 19.

4. Macules with or without blisters with irregular shape and size. See Fig. 20.

Figures 17-20 are *examples* of the described lesions. However, atypical targets and macules may have morphologies that are not identical to these examples. For example, the center of an atypical target may be lighter or darker than the periphery (*Ibid.*).

Erythema multiforme minor, characterized by target lesions without epidermal detachment and without mucosal involvement, has been associated with drugs, but more often with recent herpes simplex virus infection.

EM major (Stevens-Johnson syndrome) is characterized by cutaneous lesions as described above plus mucosal erosions at two sites. (The eyes are usually affected.) See Table 8.

Blistering may occur in some lesions and may, rarely, progress and generalize over 1 to 14 days. It has been proposed that EM major (Stevens-Johnson syndrome) be defined as less than 10% epidermal detachment with widespread macules or flat atypical targets, and mucosal involvement (*Ibid.*). See Fig. 21 and Table 8.

DIFFERENTIAL DIAGNOSIS

Toxic epidermal necrolysis (only in the presence of widespread blistering and a positive Nikolsky's sign).

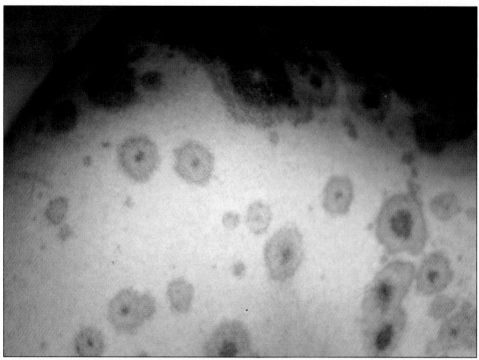

Figure 17. Typical bull's-eye and target lesions of erythema multiforme.

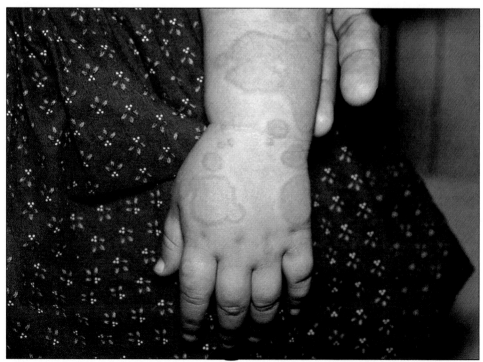

Figure 18. Raised atypical target lesions of erythema multiforme.

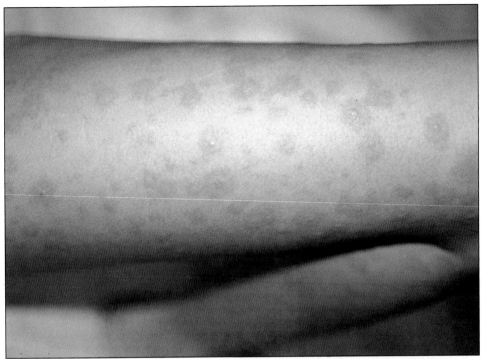

Figure 19. Flat atypical targets with round lesions reminiscent of erythema multiforme but with two zones and poorly defined border.

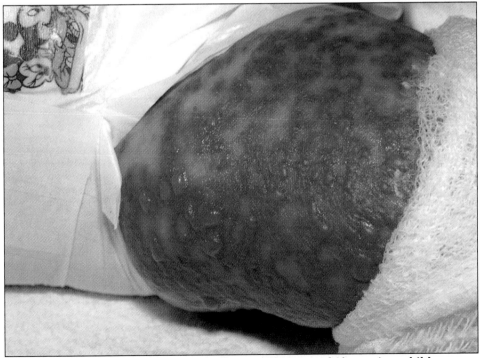

Figure 20. Macules with blisters: bullous erythema multiforme in a child treated with phenobarbital.

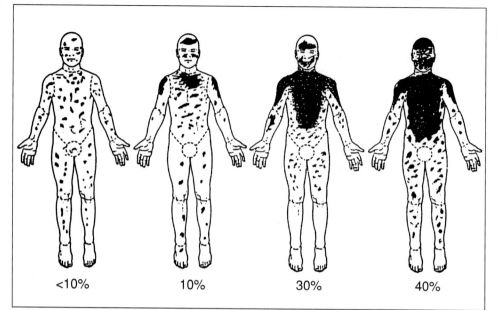

| <10% | 10% | 30% | 40% |

Figure 21. Schematic examples of the usual distribution of detachment in Stevens-Johnson syndrome—toxic epidermal necrolysis. Below 10%, sparse nonconfluent lesions; 10%, areas of confluence limited to the chest, upper back, arms and face; 30%, large areas of epidermal separation on the trunk, arms and forearms with sparse lesions elsewhere; 40%, most of the trunk is involved with minor lesions elsewhere.

Reprinted with permission from *Arch Dermatol.* 1993; 129:92-96, Copyright 1993, American Medical Association, Bastuji-Garin S, Rzany B, Stern RS, Shear NH, Naldi L, Roujeau JC. Clinical classification of cases of toxic epidermal necrolysis, Stevens-Johnson syndrome, and erythema multiforme.

TABLE 8. PROPOSED CLASSIFICATION OF CASES IN THE SPECTRUM OF SEVERE BULLOUS EM.*

Classification	Bullous EM	SJS	Overlap SJS-TEN	TEN With Spots	TEN Without Spots
Detachment	<10%	<10%	10%-30%	>30%	>10%
Typical targets	Yes	. . .	. . .	. . .	. . .
Atypical targets	Raised	Flat	Flat	Flat	. . .
Spots	. . .	Yes	Yes	Yes	. . .

* EM indicates erythema multiforme; SJS, Stevens-Johnson syndrome; and TEN, toxic epidermal necrolysis.

Reprinted with permission from *Arch Dermatol.* 1993; 129:92-96, Copyright 1993, American Medical Association, Bastuji-Garin S, Rzany B, Stern RS, Shear NH, Naldi L, Roujeau JC. Clinical classification of cases of toxic epidermal necrolysis, Stevens-Johnson syndrome, and erythema multiforme.

LABS

Skin biopsy may be helpful.

MANAGEMENT

The use of systemic steroids is controversial. Such therapy, if used, should be started early in the course before significant blistering is seen, and at high dose or at pulse therapy with appropriate caution.* Therapy should be stopped after several days if no response is noted.

Supportive care, local skin care.

Ophthalmologic consultation.

Oral care (viscous xylocaine and other preparations as needed).

Hospitalization for failure to maintain hydration or failure to urinate due to pain. Burn unit for extensive blistering.

DRUGS THAT HAVE BEEN MOST OFTEN ASSOCIATED WITH EM MAJOR

> Allopurinol
>
> Anticonvulsants - phenytoin (diphenylhydantoin)
>
> Barbiturates
>
> Carbamazepine
>
> Estrogens/progestins
>
> Gold
>
> Nonsteroidal antiinflammatory drugs
>
> Penicillamine
>
> Sulfonamides and other antibiotics

* Renfro L, Grant-Kels JM, Feder HM, et al. Controversy: are systemic steroids indicated in the treatment of erythema multiforme? *Pediatric Dermatol.* 1989; 6:43-50.

OTHER DRUGS ASSOCIATED WITH EM MAJOR

Amoxicillin
Ampicillin
Aspirin
Atropine
Cefazolin
Cephalexin
Chloral hydrate
Chloramphenicol
Chlormezanone
Clindamycin
Codeine
Diclofenac
Didanosine (ddl)
Diflunisal
Digoxin
Diltiazem
Ethosuximide
Etodolac
Etoposide
Fansidar
Fluconazole
Glutethimide
Griseofulvin
Hydralazine
Hydrochlorothiazide
Ibuprofen
Meclofenamate
Meprobamate
Methaqualone

Minocycline
Minoxidil
Nifedipine
Norfloxacin
Nystatin
Penicillins
Pentamidine (IV)
Phenobarbital
Phensuximide
Phenytoin (diphenylhydantoin)
Piroxicam
Quinine
Streptomycin
Sulfadiazine
Sulfasalazine
Sulindac
Tetracyclines
Theophylline
Thiabendazole
Thiacetazone
Thiopental
Trimethoprim
Trimethoprim +
Sulfamethoxazole
Vaccine: DTP
Vaccine: Measles
Vancomycin
Verapamil
Zidovudine

EXFOLIATIVE ERYTHRODERMA

DESCRIPTION

Generalized redness and scaling over the entire body surface, except palms and soles.

Patient often shivers and may be febrile.

Blisters are not part of the presentation.

High output cardiac failure may rarely occur.

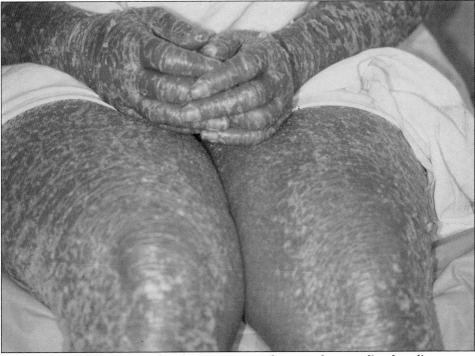

Figure 22. Exfoliative erythroderma. Note redness and generalized scaling.

DIFFERENTIAL DIAGNOSIS

The following may have erythrodermic stages:

Psoriasis.

Atopic dermatitis.

Contact dermatitis.

Seborrheic dermatitis.

Cutaneous T cell lymphoma (Sezary syndrome).

LABS

Skin biopsy may reveal T cell lymphoma, but may be nonspecific and not diagnostic of an underlying cause during the initial presentation.

A Sezary preparation of white blood cells may suggest cutaneous T cell lymphoma. T cell receptor gene rearrangement studies on peripheral WBC may be more sensitive than Sezary preparations.

MANAGEMENT

Treatment with wet compresses and topical steroids initially.

Further treatment is based on determination of the underlying cause.

DRUGS COMMONLY ASSOCIATED WITH EXFOLIATIVE ERYTHRODERMA

Barbiturates

Captopril

Carbamazepine

Cimetidine

Furosemide

Gold

Isoniazid (INH)

Lithium

Nonsteroidal antiinflammatory drugs

Penicillamine

Phenytoin (diphenylhydantoin)

Quinidine

Sulfas

Thiazides

OTHER DRUGS ASSOCIATED WITH EXFOLIATIVE ERYTHRODERMA

Allopurinol
Aminoglutethimide
Aminophylline
Amiodarone
Amitriptyline
Amoxicillin
Ampicillin
Arsenic
Aspirin
Atropine
Aztreonam
Bacampicillin
Benzathine penicillin
Bumetanide
Cefoxitin
Chloroquine
Chlorpromazine
Chlorpropamide
Chlortetracycline
Codeine
Dactinomycin
Dapsone
Diclofenac
Diflunisal
Diltiazem
Doxycycline
Ethambutol
Etodolac
Fenoprofen
Fluphenazine
Flurbiprofen
Griseofulvin
Hydroxychloroquine
Ibuprofen
Imipramine
Iodine
Isosorbide dinitrate
Ketoconazole

Ketoprofen
Lincomycin
Meclofenamate
Mephenytoin
Meprobamate
Mercury
Methotrexate
Minocycline
Nifedipine
Nitrofurantoin
Nitroglycerin
Nizatidine
Norfloxacin
Paramethadione
Penicillins
Pentobarbital
Perphenazine
Phenobarbital
Phenolphthalein
Piroxicam
Primodone
Quinacrine
Rifampin
Streptomycin
Sulfadoxine
Sulfamethoxazole
Sulfasalazine
Sulfisoxazole
Sulindac
Tetracycline
Thiethylperazine
Thioridazine
Thiothixene
Tobramycin
Trimethadione
Trimethoprim + Sulfamethoxazole
Vaccine: Measles
Vancomycin

HYPERSENSITIVITY VASCULITIS

(PALPABLE PURPURA; LEUKOCYTOCLASTIC VASCULITIS; NECROTIZING VENULITIS/ANGIITIS)

DESCRIPTION

Small (one to a few mm) purpuric papules ("palpable purpura") and occasional hemorrhagic vesicles.

Lesions may appear raised only on side-lighting and not by palpation.

Often limited to or most prominent on the lower extremities.

Vasculitis can also present as macules, papules, urticarial lesions and bullae.

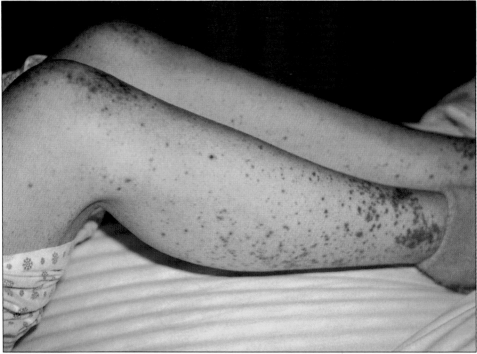

Figure 23. Palpable purpura due to nafcillin. Biopsy revealed leukocytoclastic vasculitis.

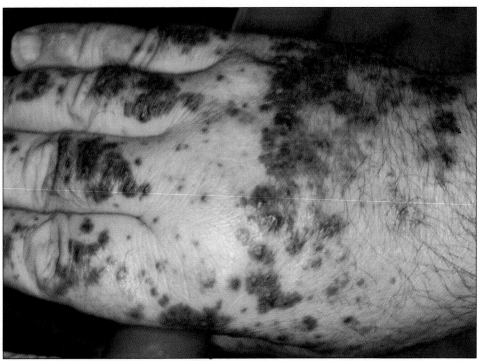

Figure 24. Purpuric plaques and hemorrhagic vesicles on the hand due to nafcillin.

Differential diagnosis

First look elsewhere, and distinguish between true palpable purpura, and a nonvasculitic rash that is purpuric only on the lower extremities. Purpura may occasionally occur in inflammatory rashes on the legs from extravasation of red blood cells from small vessels surrounded by an inflammatory infiltrate.

Petechiae should not be raised.

Pigmenting purpura (several clinical variants including Schamberg's disease), an innocuous capillaritis with brown macules interspersed with tiny (< 1 mm) red "cayenne pepper"-colored macules on the lower legs.

Schönlein-Henoch purpura in children associated with diffuse abdominal pain or bowel ischemia (vasculitis with IgA deposits in skin); clinically, may have an appearance identical to hypersensitivity vasculitis, or may present with crusted hemorrhagic plaques.

Etiology

Necrotizing vasculitis may be caused by drugs or infection, or may be associated with cryoproteins, collagen vascular disease or malignancy.

LABS

Skin biopsy is essential to establish the diagnosis, followed by cryoproteins, CBC, and workup for infection as clinically indicated, to determine the cause. Direct immunofluorescence on new lesions may disclose IgA in blood vessel walls in Henoch-Schoenlein purpura.

The main reason for making the diagnosis is to rule out vasculitis in other organ systems, and a stool guaiac and urinalysis may be indicated.

MANAGEMENT

Cessation of drug. Pharmacologic treatment (e.g., antihistamines, colchicine, prednisone) is often not needed.

DRUGS COMMONLY ASSOCIATED WITH HYPERSENSITIVITY VASCULITIS

Allopurinol
Animal antisera
Antibiotics
Furosemide
Gold
Nonsteroidal antiinflammatory drugs
Phenytoin (diphenylhydantoin)
Thiazides

OTHER DRUGS THAT MAY CAUSE HYPERSENSITIVITY VASCULITIS

Amiodarone
Amitriptyline
Amphetamine
Ampicillin
Antithymocyte globulin
Arsenic
Aspirin
Atenolol
Atropine
Azathioprine
BCG (Bacille Calmette-Guerin)
Benzoic acid
Captopril
Carbamazepine
Chloramphenicol
Chloroquine
Chlorpromazine
Chlorpropamide
Chlortetracycline
Chlorthalidone
Cimetidine
Ciprofloxacin
Clindamycin
Cromolyn sodium
Cyclophosphamide
Difunisal

Diltiazem
Dimenhydrinate
Diphenhydramine
Disopyramide
Disulfiram
Enalapril
Ephedrine
Erythrityl tetranitrate
Ethacrynic acid
Etodolac
Famotidine
Fenbufen
Flurbiprofen
Furosemide
Gemfibrozil
Glyburide
Griseofulvin
Guanethidine
Hydralazine
Hydrochlorothiazide
Hydroxyurea
Ibuprofen
Indapamide
Indomethacin
Insulin
Iron (Ferrous gluconate sulfate)
Isoniazid (INH)
Isosorbide
Isotretinoin
Labetalol
Levamisole
Lithium
Lisinopril
Lovastatin
Maprotiline
Meclofenamate
Mefenamic acid
Melphalan
Methotrexate
Methylphenidate
Metolazone
Naproxen

Ofloxacin
Oral contraceptive agents
Oxytetracycline
Penicillamine
Penicillins
Pentamidine (IV)
Phenobarbital
Phenytoin (diphenylhydantoin)
Pindolol
Piroxicam
Procainamide
Propylthiouracil
Quinethazone
Quinidine
Radiographic contrast media
Ranitidine
Rifampin
Spironolactone
Streptokinase
Streptomycin
Sulfasalazine
Sulfisoxazole
Sulindac
Tamoxifen
Tartrazine
Terbutaline
Tetracycline
Thiazide derivatives
Ticlopidine
Tiopronin
Trimethoprim + Sulfamethoxazole
Vaccine: BCG (S.3.14d)
Vaccine: Influenza
Vaccine: Poliomyelitis (Salk)
Vaccine: Rabies
Vaccine: Rubella
Valproic acid
Vancomycin
Verapamil
Vitamin B6 (Pyridoxine)
Zidovudine

ERYTHEMA NODOSUM

DESCRIPTION

Tender red subcutaneous nodules.

Most commonly occurs on the shins, but may appear on other areas such as the thighs.

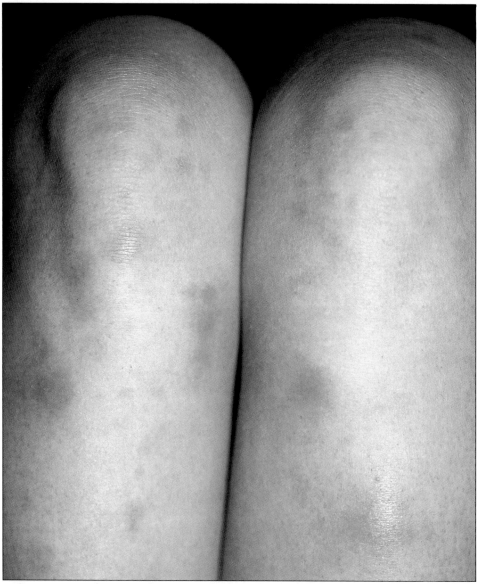

Figure 25. Erythema nodosum on the lower extremities.

DIFFERENTIAL DIAGNOSIS

Red nodules may be caused by various forms of panniculitis, fat necrosis, infection, systemic vasculitis, trauma and phlebitis.

Erythema nodosum may be associated with infection (e.g., streptococcal, viral, coccidiomycosis, tuberculosis), sarcoidosis, malignancies, enteropathies.

LABS

Adequate biopsy of early lesions can be definitive, but may not always be required in the presence of a classic presentation.

Workup for infection as clinically indicated.

MANAGEMENT

Treat underlying conditions.

Use of nonsteroidal antiinflammatory agents or potassium iodide to control the skin lesions as needed.

DRUGS MOST COMMONLY ASSOCIATED WITH ERYTHEMA NODOSUM

Antibiotics

Amiodarone

Estrogens/progestins

Gold

Nonsteroidal antiinflammatory drugs

Opiates

OTHER DRUGS THAT MAY CAUSE ERYTHEMA NODOSUM

Antipyrine

Arsenic

Aspirin

Barbiturates

Benzathine penicillin

Bromine

Busulfan

Carbamazepine

Chlordiazepoxide

Chlorotrianisene

Chlorpropamide

Ciprofloxacin

Codeine

Dapsone

Diclofenac

Diethylstilbestrol

Estrogens

Ethinyl estradiol +
Ethynodiol diacetate

Ethinyl estradiol +
Megestrol acetate

Ethinyl estradiol +
Norgestrel

Hydralazine

Indomethacin

Interleukin 2

Iodine

Isotretinoin

Levamisole

Levonorgestrel

Loperamide

Meclofenamate

Meprobamate

Mestranol

Mestranol + Norethindrone

Minocycline

Nifedipine

Nitrofurantoin

Oral contraceptives

Penicillamine

Penicillins

Phenobarbital

Prazosin

Pyritinol

Quinestrol

Streptomycin

Sulfamethoxazole

Sulfamethoxypyridazine

Sulfanilamide

Sulfathiazole

Tolbutamide

Trimethoprim

Vaccine: BCG

Vaccine: DTP

Vaccine: Poliomyelitis (Salk)

Vaccine: Tetanus antitoxin

Vitamin D

ACNEIFORM ERUPTION

DESCRIPTION

New onset or worsening of acne-like lesions.

Located on head, upper trunk, and upper extremities.

Lesions of steroid "acne" consist of monomorphic, follicular papules and pustules.

Comedones are not associated with systemic drugs except halogenated aromatic hydrocarbons (chloracne).

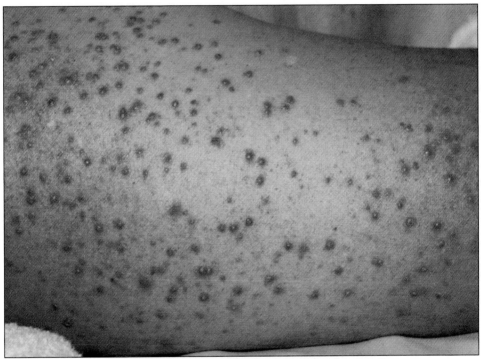

Figure 26. Acne-like eruption on arm during tapering of systemic corticosteroids.

Differential diagnosis

Acne vulgaris.
Folliculitis (bacterial and nonbacterial).

Labs

Usually not helpful.

Treatment

Discontinue exposure.
Antiacne medications may be of benefit.

Drugs that may cause an acneiform eruption

ACTH (Adrenocorticotropic Hormone)
Androgens
Bromides
Corticosteroids
Halothane
Iodides
Isoniazid (INH)
Lithium
Phenytoin (diphenylhydantoin)
Vitamins B2, B6, B12

OTHER DRUGS THAT MAY CAUSE ACNEIFORM ERUPTIONS

Allopurinol
Amphetamine
Azathioprine
Barbiturates
Bromine
Chloral hydrate
Chloroquine
Cimetidine
Ciprofloxacin
Clofazimine
Cyclophosphamide
Cyclosporine A
Dactinomycin
Danazol
Dantrolene
Dexamethasone
Diazepam
Diclofenac
Disulfiram
Erythromycin
Erythropoietin
Estrogens
Ethionamide
Fenoprofen
Fluoxymesterone
Folic acid
Gold
Haloperidol
Hydantoin
Hydrocortisone
Interferon a 2b

Iodine
Mercury
Methamphetamine
Methotrexate
Methoxsalen plus UV light (PUVA)
Methylprednisolone
Naproxen
Nonsteroidal antiinflammatory drugs
Nystatin
Oral contraceptives
Paramethadione
Penicillins
Phenobarbital
Piroxicam
Prednisone
Progesterone derivatives
Propranolol
Quinidine
Quinine
Rifampin
Salicylates
Streptomycin
Testosterone
Tetracycline
Triamcinolone
Trimethadione
Vinblastine
Vitamin A
Vitamin D
Zidovudine

HYPERTRICHOSIS/HIRSUTISM

DESCRIPTION

Hypertrichosis refers to the appearance of increased or coarser hair in nonsexually determined areas (i.e., other than scalp/beard/escutcheon, that are affected in hirsutism).

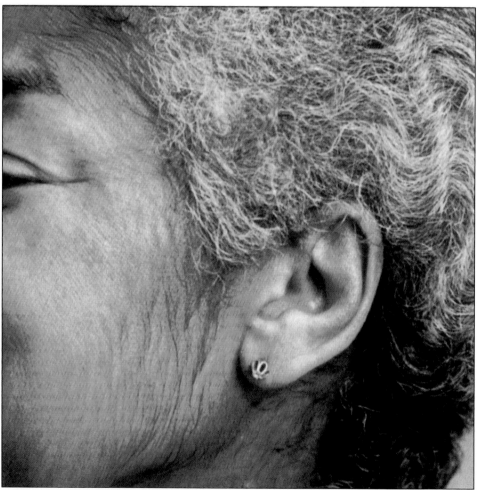

Figure 27. Hypertrichosis due to orally administered minoxidil.

LABS

Androgen levels are often indicated in hirsutism, not hypertrichosis.

MANAGEMENT

Discontinuation of drug often results in at least partial reversal of hypertrichosis over many months.

DRUGS ASSOCIATED WITH HYPERTRICHOSIS

Corticosteroids
Diazoxide
Minoxidil
Phenytoin (diphenylhydantoin)

OTHER DRUGS ASSOCIATED WITH HYPERTRICHOSIS

ACTH (Adrenocorticotropic Hormone)
Amantadine
Amiodarone
Chlorpromazine
Cyclosporine A
Dexamethasone
Diazoxide
Diethylstilbestrol
Estrogens
Hydrocortisone
Interferon alpha (2a or 2b)
Isoniazid (INH)
Isotretinoin
Methoxsalen plus UV light (PUVA)
Nystatin
Oral contraceptives
Penicillamine
Streptomycin
Triamcinolone
Valproic acid
Zidovudine

DRUGS REPORTED TO CAUSE HIRSUTISM

Acetazolamide

ACTH (Adrenocorticotropic Hormone)

Androgens

Chlorotrianisene

Clonazepam

Corticosteroids

Danazol

Dexamethasone

Diazoxide

Diethylstilbestrol

Estrogens

Ethosuximide

Fluoxymesterone

Levonorgestrel

Mestranol + Norethindrone

Minoxidil

Oral contraceptives

Oxymetholone

Penicillamine

Phenytoin (diphenylhydantoin)

Progesterone derivatives

Quinestrol

Spironolactone

Testosterone

Thioridazine

Triamcinolone

DRUG-INDUCED ALOPECIA

DESCRIPTION

Onset of loss of hair or hair thinning, often in a diffuse pattern.

May be due to interruption of the anagen cycle of hair (with chemotherapeutic agents) or other mechanisms such as telogen effluvium.

The scalp itself is usually normal.

Sites other than the scalp may be involved.

DIFFERENTIAL DIAGNOSIS

Endocrinopathy.

Androgenetic alopecia (so-called male pattern baldness).

Telogen effluvium, after crash dieting, fever, childbirth, shock, etc., that cause a higher percent of hairs to go into resting (telogen) phase. Increased hair shedding begins a few months later when new hairs begin to grow again, pushing the old telogen hairs out.

LABS

In patients with telogen effluvium, and alopecia areata, gentle tugging of the hair will often dislodge more than 6 telogen hairs (with small white bulbs). In contrast, in chemotherapy-induced alopecia, 90% of the hairs break on tugging, leaving a tapered end.

A scalp biopsy, though seldom needed in the setting of drug-induced alopecia, may be helpful in ruling out other diseases, especially if two biopsies are submitted and sectioned both horizontally and vertically.

Potassium hydrochloride (KOH) preparation and fungal culture may be performed when indicated.

MANAGEMENT

Discontinue the drug when possible.

DRUGS THAT MAY CAUSE ALOPECIA

Amantadine

Androgens

Azathioprine

Bleomycin

Cimetidine

Colchicine

Cyclophosphamide

Cytarabine

Daunorubicin

Doxorubicin

Etretinate

Heavy metals

Heparin

Isotretinoin

Methotrexate

Progestins

Propranolol

Vincristine

Warfarin

Other drugs that have been reported to cause alopecia

Acetaminophen
Acyclovir
Allopurinol
Amiloride
Aminophylline
Amiodarone
Amitriptyline
Amphetamine
Antithymocyte globulin
Arsenic
Aspirin
Atenolol
BCNU (Carmustine)
Bismuth
Borate
Boric acid
Bromocriptine
Busulfan
Captopril
Carbamazepine
CCNU (Lomustine)
Chlorambucil
Chloramphenicol
Chlordiazepoxide
Chloroquine
Chlorotrianisene
Chlorpropamide
Chorionic gonadotropin (HCG)
Cisplatin
Clofibrate
Clomiphene
Clonazepam
Clonidine
Corticosteroids
Cyclosporine A
Dactinomycin
Danazol

Desipramine
Dextran
Diazoxide
Diclofenac
Dicumarol
Diethylstilbestrol
Disopyramide
Doxepin
Estrogens
Ethambutol
Ethinyl estradiol + Ethynodioldiacetate
Ethinyl estradiol + Megestrol acetate
Ethionamide
Etoposide
Famotidine
Fenfluramine
5-Fluorouracil
Fluoxymesterone
Flurbiprofen
Gentamicin
Gold
Griseofulvin
Guanethidine
Haloperidol
Halothane
Hydroxychloroquine
Hydroxyurea
Ibuprofen
Imipramine
Indomethacin
Interferon alpha (2a or 2b)
Interleukin 2
Iodine
Isoniazid (INH)
Ketoconazole

Ketoprofen
Labetalol
L-Asparaginase
Levamisole
Levonorgestrel
Levodopa
Levothyroxine
Lithium
Loxapine
Mechlorethamine (Mustine)
Melphalan
Mephenytoin
Mercaptopurine
Mercury
Mestranol + Norethindrone
Methamphetamine
Methimazole (thiamzole)
Methoxsalen plus UV light (PUVA)
Methyldopa
Methylphenidate
Methylprednisolone
Methysergide (Maleate)
Metoprolol tartrate
Mexiletine
Minoxidil
Mitomycin C
Nalidixic acid
Naproxen
Nicotinic acid
Nifedipine
Nitrofurantoin
Nortriptyline
Oral contraceptive agents
Paramethadione
Penicillamine

Phenobarbital
Phenolphthalein
Phensuximide
Phenytoin (diphenylhydantoin)
Piroxicam
Prazosin
Probenecid
Procarbazine
Progesterone derivatives
Propylthiouracil
Protriptyline
Pyrazinamide
Quinacrine
Quinestrol
Quinidine
Quinine
Ranitidine
Reserpine
Simvastatin
Spironolactone
Sulfasalazine
Sulindac
Tamoxifen
Taxol
Testosterone
Thallium
Thiacetazone
Thioguanine
Thiotepa
Tiopronin
Trimethadione
Valproic acid
Verapamil
Vinblastine
Vitamin A (Retinol)

HYPERPIGMENTATION

DESCRIPTION

Appearance of brown, gray or blue-black macules on skin, nails, and/or mucosa.
Pattern and color may suggest specific conditions and drugs.
May be caused by both systemic and topical drugs.

DIFFERENTIAL DIAGNOSIS

Endocrinopathies.
Postinflammatory hyperpigmentation.

LABS

Often not diagnostic. Skin biopsy may be helpful.

PROGNOSIS

Often depends on the type of drug. May be very long-lasting.

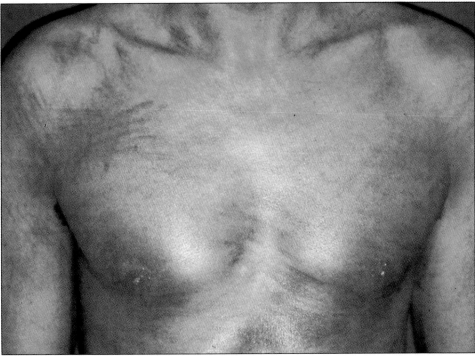

Figure 28. Hyperpigmentation due to bleomycin.

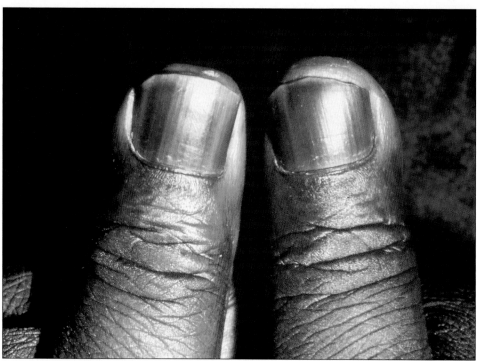

Figure 29. Hyperpigmentation of the nails due to azidothymidine.

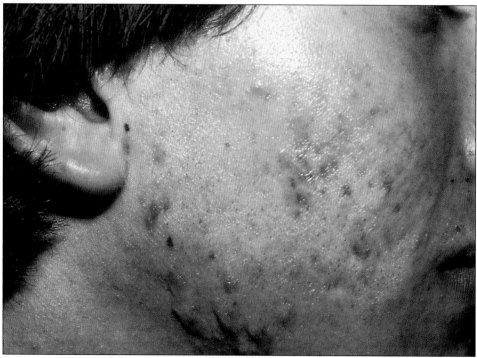

Figure 30. Hyperpigmentation due to minocycline.

TABLE 9. DRUG-INDUCED CHANGES IN SKIN COLOR.

	Color	Location
ACTH (Adrenocortico-tropic Hormone)	melasma, brown	generalized
Amiodarone	metalic-bluish, silver or slate-gray	photodistributed
Azathioprine	hypermelanosis	photodistributed, red nail lunulae: 2%
Azidothymidine (AZT) (see p. 160)	brown to blue to black	nail-bands or diffuse lunulae,
	brown	tongue, oral mucosa
	brown	diffuse, forehead, palmar-plantar
Bismuth	blue-gray	generalized/ gingival mucosa
Bleomycin	brown	streaky linear/flagellate, reticulated on trunk, in areas of pressure or scratching
Busulfan	Addisonian	also fingernails, mucous membranes rarely
Carbamazepine	(details not reported)	
Chloroquine, Hydroxychloroquine, Quinacrine	brown to black, slate gray-bluish	face and hard palate, conjunctivae, and on extremities
Chlorpromazine	brownish to bluish to slate gray	photodistributed, visceral, conjunctival, cornea, nails, nipples
Clofazimine	brown-red, ~100%	generalized conjunctivae, nails
	slate-gray	
Corticosteroids	brown	photodistributed, spots
Coumarin(s)	purple, "purple toe"	plantar, toes
Cyclophosphamide	brown	generalized, localized, palmar-plantar, nail bands photodistributed, teeth
Dapsone	blue gray with methemaglobinemia, brown	postinflammatory

TABLE 9. CONTINUED.

	Color	Location
Daunorubicin	brown	nails, palmar-plantar, photodistributed
Desipramine	slate-gray	photodistributed gold-colored irises
Diazoxide	brown	
Doxorubicin	brown	nails, palmar-plantar, dorsal finger joints, face
Estrogen	melasma, brown	areolae/nipples and vulva, genitals
Ethionamide	lilac-brown	photodistributed
5-Fluorouracil	brown, Addisonian or bluish or brown	photodistributed, nail bands
Glutethimide	brown	spots
Gold	chrysiasis: gray-brown, sometimes purple, blue-gray	generalized, photodistributed, nails
Griseofulvin	brownish	genitals, nipples
Hydrochlorothiazide	bluish-black, brown	photodistributed
Hydroxyurea	hypermelanosis, yellow-gray-brown	generalized, forehead/palmar creases
Imipramine	brown?, bluish-gray, "visage mauve"	face, throat, hands
Iron	brown in hemochromatosis	generalized
Mephenytoin	brown	melasma-like Addisonian
Mercaptopurine	brown,	Addisonian or pellagra-like
Mercury	gray	face, hands, fingernails
Methaqualon	brown	tongue
Methyldopa	brown	generalized
Methysergide	reddish, peaux d'orange	
Minocycline	blue-gray spotty or diffuse pigment	often on lower extremities/oral mucosa
	gray-brown	diffuse, photodistributed, shins

TABLE 9. CONTINUED.

	Color	Location
Nicotinic acid derivatives	brown, after long-term therapy	Acanthosis nigricans-like
Nitrofurantoin	brownish	melasma-like
Perphenazine	brownish to bluish to slate-gray	photodistributed
Phenazopyridine	yellow-orange	generalized
Phenolphthalein	dark gray	generalized, spots, nails, blue lunulae
Phenothiazines	blue-gray	photoexposed areas
Phenytoin	brown	melasma-like in women
Prochlorperazine	brownish to bluish to slate-gray	photodistributed
Progesterone	brown	melasma
Propranolol	brown	tongue
Propylthiouracil	brown	(not described)
Pyrazinamide	red-brown	photodistributed
Quinacrine	diffuse yellow color	skin, nail beds, and sclerae
Quinine	brown	generalized
Rifampicin	orange, red	
Silver	argyria, bluish-gray,	generalized, photodistributed
	blue	nails
Spironolactone	brown	gereralized/ melasma-like
Tetracycline derivatives	yellow-gray	teeth
	brownish	acne lesions
Thiabendazole	brown, spotted	generalized
Thioridazine	brownish to bluish to slate-gray	photodistributed
Vitamin A (overdose)	yellow-orange	generalized
	brown	melasma-like

HYPOPIGMENTATION

DESCRIPTION

Appearance of areas of decreased pigmentation.

Loss of pigmentation from systemically administered drugs is rarely total (i.e., depigmented or white).

Most hypopigmentation and depigmentation is due to topically used drugs and other agents.

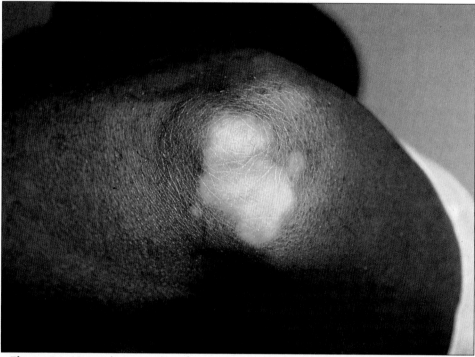

Figure 31. Hypopigmentation due to an intralesional injection of triamcinolone.

DIFFERENTIAL DIAGNOSIS

Vitiligo, marked by depigmentation.

Postinflammatory hypopigmentation.

LABS

Not helpful.

MANAGEMENT

Discontinuation of drug.

Await spontaneous repigmentation in many cases.

DRUGS THAT MAY CAUSE HYPOPIGMENTATION

Systemically administered drugs rarely cause hypopigmentation except for the metals arsenic and mercury, and chloroquine, quinacrine, thiotepa (palpebral changes) interferon α 2b, penicillamine and etretinate.

Topically applied agents may cause hypopigmentation and include:

Hydroquinone and monobenzylether of hydroquinone (the latter causes permanent depigmentation).

Corticosteroids (particularly if injected intralesionally), 5-fluorouracil and tretinoin.

CHEMOTHERAPY-ASSOCIATED PALMAR-PLANTAR ERYTHRODYSESTHESIA SYNDROME (ACRAL ERYTHEMA)

DESCRIPTION

Dysesthesia and pain evolving over 3 to 4 days, with periungual erythema and symmetric swelling and redness of the distal phalanges.

Bullous formation and sloughing may occur rarely. A recent report suggests that this progression may be associated more with cytarabine, and not 5-fluorouracil or doxorubicin (Waltzer JF, Flowers FP 1993). There is a possible association of acral erythema with pericardial and pleural effusions (Vukelja SJ, Sharkey HJ, et al 1993).

Resolves over 5 to 7 days with desquamation on discontinuation of therapy.

DIAGNOSIS

Clinical correlation.

One reported case had typical palmar lesions, with a biopsy that demonstrated necrotizing eccrine squamous syringometaplasia, which is thought to be a clinical and pathologic entity distinct from acral erythema, although both may represent cytotoxic reactions (Rongioletti F, Ballestrero A, Bogliolo F, et al 1991).

DRUGS

5-Fluorouracil, cytarabine, doxorubicin usually administered by continuous intravenous infusion, cyclophosphamide, methotrexate, mercaptopurine.

MECHANISM

Cytotoxicity.

MANAGEMENT

Cessation of continuous drug infusion.

Cool compresses. Topical steroids are of limited benefit.

NEUTROPHILIC ECCRINE HIDRADENITIS

DESCRIPTION

Onset of tender violaceous or red papules, nodules or plaques, or patches of diffuse hyperpigmentation.

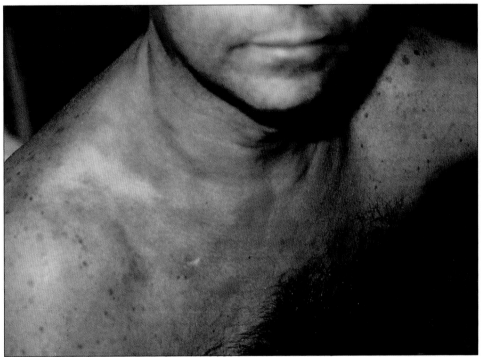

Figure 32. Neutrophilic eccrine hidradenitis. Reprinted with permission from Cutis (1991; 48:198-200). Courtesy of Dr. David J. Margolis and Dr. Paul R. Gross.

LOCATION

Upper trunk and extremities, face and palms.

DIAGNOSIS

Skin biopsy with tissue gram stain and culture of the biopsy specimen.

DIFFERENTIAL DIAGNOSIS

Syringosquamous metaplasia (also called eccrine squamous syringometaplasia) is an entity thought to be related clinically and histopathologically to neutrophilic eccrine hidradenitis. Patients present with small erythematous papules and plaques, most often after treatment with cytarabine, although multiple chemotherapeutic agents have been used in patients with this reaction pattern. It is thought that this might represent a cytotoxic reaction. Diagnosis is established by skin biopsy.

DRUGS

Cancer chemotherapeutic agents: bleomycin and cytarabine; zidovudine (AZT); acetaminophen.

OTHER CAUSES

Has been associated with infection (*Enterobacter, Serratia*).

MANAGEMENT

Continue chemotherapy. Treat infection as indicated. May or may not recur on repeat courses of treatment.

VITAMIN K HYPERSENSITIVITY

DESCRIPTION

Appearance of red indurated plaques or eczematous areas, often with pruritus, at sites of injection of oil-soluble vitamin K_1. Large patches of erythema and a morbilliform rash are occasionally seen.

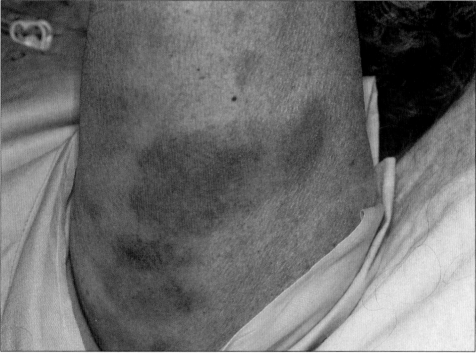

Figure 33. Plaque due to vitamin K hypersensitivity.

ONSET

2-14 days after injection.

MECHANISM

Patch and intradermal skin testing suggest Type IV hypersensitivity to vitamin K_1 and occasionally to vitamin K_2.

DIAGNOSIS

Clinical. Skin biopsy may be helpful.

MANAGEMENT

Use of topical steroids and substitution of vitamin K_3 for vitamin K_1.

PROGNOSIS

Usually resolves in weeks or months; the area may become sclerotic, however.

ALLOPURINOL TOXICITY (HYPERSENSITIVITY) SYNDROME

DESCRIPTION

Syndrome of widespread maculopapular eruption or exfoliative erythroderma with fever, hepatitis, eosinophilia, and worsening renal function. TEN and erythema multiforme major also noted.

ONSET

Usually within the first month of therapy.

MECHANISM

Almost all patients have preexistent renal insufficiency. It is thought that high levels of allopurinol or metabolites may cause vasculitis or a hypersensitivity reaction.

DIAGNOSIS

Clinical picture plus liver and renal function tests.

MANAGEMENT

Discontinuation of allopurinol, hemodialysis, and use of systemic corticosteroids.

PREVENTION

Use of reduced dosages in patients with renal insufficiency.

PROGNOSIS

Rapid or gradual clearing, at times over months. May be fatal. Some patients show recurrence on rechallenge. In others, drug may be introduced at very low doses and gradually increased.

NOTE ON HYPERSENSITIVITY SYNDROMES

Several drugs, including phenytoin, dapsone and sulfas, also may cause hypersensitivity syndromes, characterized by fever, often with skin rash, hepatic abnormalities, leukocytosis with eosinophilia, lymphadenopathy, and occasionally with renal and CNS involvement. Although thought to be due to toxic metabolites, the pathogenesis of these syndromes is unclear.

LUPUS ERYTHEMATOSUS-LIKE REACTIONS

DESCRIPTION

Onset of polyarthritis, pleuritis, pneumonitis, fever and myalgias. CNS and renal involvement are rare. Typically, the patient is older than a patient with idiopathic LE, and less often African-American. Males are affected slightly more often than females.

Skin lesions are less common than in idiopathic systemic lupus erythematosus (SLE), and usually not of the scarring "discoid" LE type. It may be difficult to distinguish between idiopathic and drug-associated LE on clinical grounds alone.

Drug-induced lupus-like reactions are often dose-related. Often, only serologic abnormalities (positive ANA) are seen.

It is unclear in what percent of patients a drug unmasks a genetic predisposition to LE.

ONSET

Variable, from months to years.

DIAGNOSIS

Clinical, combined with response to discontinuation of drug. Antihistone Antinuclear Antibody (ANA) and antileukocyte ANA are often positive, and anti-double-stranded-DNA antibodies are often negative in LE-like reactions. ANA (diffuse pattern) may be positive in drug-related or idiopathic LE. Direct skin immunofluorescence studies are often negative in drug-associated LE reactions.

PROGNOSIS

Clinical signs should resolve on discontinuation of medication. Serologies resolve more slowly.

DRUGS MOST COMMONLY ASSOCIATED WITH LUPUS ERYTHEMATOSUS-LIKE REACTIONS

Carbamazepine

Chlorpromazine

Hydralazine

Isoniazid (INH)

Lithium

Methyldopa

Minoxidil

Oral contraceptives

Penicillamine

Phenytoin (diphenylhydantoin)

Procainamide

Propylthiouracil

Quinidine

TABLE 10. DRUG-INDUCED LUPUS ERYTHEMATOSUS.

	Induction of systemic lupus or LE-like syndrome	Aggravation of preexisting SLE or cutaneous LE	Induction of cutaneous LE	Serologic abnormalities only
Allopurinol		+		
Aminophylline		+?		
Ampicillin				+
Carbamazepine	+	+	+?	+
Cefalothin	+?			
Chlordiazepoxide	+?		+	
Chloroquine		+		
Chlorpromazine	+	+	+	+
Chlorpropamide	+?			
Chlorprothixene	+		+	
Clofibrate	+?			
Corticosteroids	+	+?	+?	
Cromolyn sodium	+			
Dapsone		+	+	
Disulfiram				
Estrogen	+	+?		+
Ethambutol	+			
Ethionamide			+	
Ethosuximide	+			
Glutethimide	+?			
Gold derivative	+	+		
Griseofulvin	+	+	+	+
Hydralazine	+		+	+
Ibuprofen	+	+		
Imipramine			+?	
Isoniazid (INH)	+		+	+
Levodopa				+
Lithium		+	+	+
Lovastatin	+			+
Meprobamate		+		

TABLE 10. CONTINUED.

	Induction of systemic lupus or LE-like syndrome	Aggravation of preexisting SLE or cutaneous LE	Induction of cutaneous LE	Serologic abnormalities only
Mercaptopurine	+			
Methamphetamine				
Methoxsalen + UVA=PUVA			+	+
Methyldopa	+			+
Methylsergide		+	+	
Nalidixic acid	+	+?		
Nitrofurantoin	+			+
Penicillamine	+		+	+
Penicillin	+	+	+	+
Perphenazine	+?		+	+
Phenelzine	+			
Phenolphthalein	+?	+		
Phenytoin (diphenylhydantoin)		+		+
Piroxicam		+		+
Primodone	+			
Procainamide	+		+	+
Prochlorperazine			+	
Promethazine	+?	+		+
Propranolol	+			
Quinidine	+		+	+
Quinine	+	+?		+
Rifampicin	+?		+	
Streptomycin	+	+		
Sulfonamide Derivatives	+	+	+	
Tetanus-Antitoxin	+?			
Tetracycline	+?	+	+	+
Thioridazine	+		+	+?
Tolbutamide		+		

COUMARIN NECROSIS

DESCRIPTION

Appearance of tender ecchymotic areas that progress to hemorrhagic blisters on buttocks, breasts, thighs and lower extremities. Necrosis and eschar formation follow.

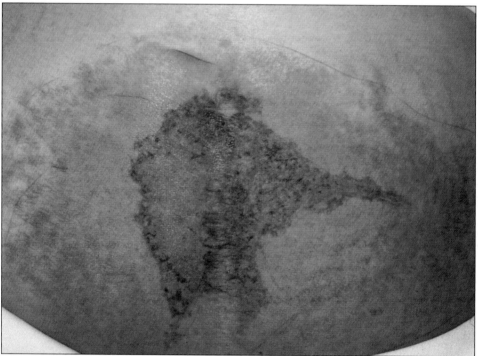

Figure 34. Coumarin necrosis on the lower abdomen.

ONSET

Often within the first week of administration.

DIAGNOSIS

Clinical. Early skin biopsy may be suggestive.

MECHANISM

Protein C deficiency may be involved. See p.103.

MANAGEMENT

Debridement and local care.

ACUTE GENERALIZED EXANTHEMATOUS PUSTULOSIS

DESCRIPTION

A widespread edematous scarlatiniform rash covered with dozens of nonfollicular small pustules on an edematous red base.* Arises on the face or intertriginous areas, and spreads over hours. Facial edema, purpura, target lesions, vesicles or blisters, as well as oral erosions may occur. Arthritis was not noted. Temperature above 38°C, leukocytosis with eosinophilia peaking on day 4 and lasting for 12 days, mild hypocalcemia, and mild transient decreases in creatinine clearance were also noted.

HISTOPATHOLOGY

One or more of the following: Spongiform superficial pustules, papillary edema, or polymorphous perivascular infiltrates with eosinophils. In many cases the epidermis showed spongiosis or was normal; focal keratinocyte necrosis was uncommon, as was leukocytoclastic vasculitis.

ONSET

Often within 24 hours of drug exposure, with a mean of 5 days.

MECHANISM

Unknown. A minority of patients have a history of plaque-type psoriasis. Some may have active enterovirus infections.

DIAGNOSIS

Clinical picture plus histopathology. Cultures are usually negative for pathogens.

*Roujeau JC, Bioulac-Sage P, Bourseau C, et al. Acute generalized exanthematous pustulosis. Analysis of 63 cases. *Arch Dermatol.* 1991; 127:1333-1338.

DIFFERENTIAL DIAGNOSIS

Pustular psoriasis, Sweet's syndrome, necrotizing vasculitis.

CAUSATIVE AGENTS[*]

Nonsulfa antibiotics are the most common cause.
Acetaminophen
Amoxicillin
Ampicillin
Carbamazepine
Erythromycin
Nifedipine
Penicillin
Quinidine
Vancomycin

PROGNOSIS

Spontaneous resolution over two weeks.

*Roujeau JC, Bioulac-Sage P, Bourseau C, et al. Acute generalized exanthematous pustulosis. Analysis of 63 cases. *Arch Dermatol.* 1991; 127:1333-1338.

THE CUTANEOUS ERUPTION OF LYMPHOCYTE RECOVERY (ELR)

DESCRIPTION

Red, morbilliform or maculopapular rash, often with fever of up to 40°C, in patients with leukemia who are being treated with chemotherapy. The rash may be pruritic, and may preceed the fever by several days. The eruption resolves in several days to several weeks, and may leave post inflammatory hyperpigmentation.

ONSET

Tends to begin between days 15 and 20 of inducton chemotherapy, at the time of initial recovery of peripheral lymphocyte counts. The WBC counts then often drop transiently after the onset of the rash, before eventual recovery.

HISTOPATHOLOGY

The changes are mild and not specific, although they are suggestive of the diagnosis. A mild superficial, perivascular, predominantly T lymphocyte infiltrate is seen, with slight basal vacuolization, intercellular edema, keratinocyte atypia, and rare dyskeratotic keratinocytes.* In a blind review of the histopathology of this eruption and that of graft vs host disease in patients who received autologous/syngeneic bone marrow transplants, enough dyskeratotic cells were present in 40% of the specimens from patients with the cutaneous eruption of lymphocyte recovery (ELR) to lead to an erroneous diagnosis of graft vs host disease. The histologic picture can also suggest an interpretation of spongiotic dermatitis or interface dermatitis (basal vacuolization and dyskeratosis without a lichenoid infiltrate).

* Horn TD, Redd JV et al. Cutaneous eruptions of lymphocyte recovery. *Arch Dermatol* 1989; 125:1512-1517.

DIAGNOSIS

Clinical context: the presentation of an exanthem in leukemic patients as their leukopenia begins to resolve. Skin biopsy can be consistent but not diagnostic of ELR. Skin biopsy cannot reliably distinguish between ELR and autologous graft vs host disease.*

DIFFERENTIAL DIAGNOSIS

Morbilliform drug reaction. Graft vs host disease. Viral exanthem. The clinical situation should help distinguish among these.

CAUSATIVE AGENTS

Patients had been treated with cytarabine, daunorubicin, amsacrine, etoposide, cyclophosphamide and vincristine, always in combination of two or more drugs.

MECHANISM

Unknown. While this could be a manifestation of drug hypersensitivity, there is no clearcut association with specific agents, and the eruption resolves despite their continuation.** It has been postulated that the actual return of uniquely reactive lymphocytes to the skin may cause the eruption through release of cytokines or changes in the local "immunologic milieu," or by other mechanisms.*

MANAGEMENT

Supportive. Rash resolves without intervention.

---

* Bauer DJ, Hood AF, and Horn TD. Histologic comparison of autologous graft-vs-host reaction and cutaneous eruption of lymphocyte recovery. *Arch Dermatol* 1993; 129:855-858.
** Horn TD, Redd JV et al. Cutaneous eruptions of lymphocyte recovery.
 Arch Dermatol 1989; 125:1512-1517.

ADVERSE REACTIONS AT SITES OF DRUG INJECTIONS

TABLE 11. ADVERSE REACTIONS AT SITES OF DRUG INJECTIONS.

Drug	Reaction
Vitamin K	Inflamed plaques, localized scleroderma.
Corticosteroids	Hemorrhage, dermal atrophy, pigmentation, panniculitis, hypertrichosis, lipoatrophy.
Insulin	Fat hypertrophy, lipoatrophy or lipohypertrophy, fascial cicatrix, mesenchymoma.
Heparin	Hematoma, infection, necrosis, red plaques and patches.
Iron	Pain, brown discoloration.
Penicillin	Atrophy, necrosis, wheals.
Pentazocine	Nodules, sclerosis, ulceration, hyperpigmentation.
Morphine	Panniculitis.
Heroin/quinine	Necrotic ulceration, thrombophlebitis, cellulitis, punctate and linear scars.
Cocaine	Painful nodules, chronic edema.
Barbiturates	Ulceration.
Methamphetamine	Granulomas, hyperpigmentation, scar, slough.
Meperidine	Panniculitis, scleroderma-like lesions, wheal and flare over vein.
Antibiotics	Chronic granulomas, gluteal fibrosis.

Reprinted with permission from Robison JW, Odom RB. Delayed cutaneous reaction to phytonadione. *Arch Dermatol.* 1978; 114:1790-1792.

Note: Many other drugs cause pain on infusion or injection, or will induce inflammation or skin necrosis, if extravasated into tissue . See Zürcher K, Krebs A. *Cutaneous drug reactions.* Basel, Switzerland: S. Karger AG; 1992.

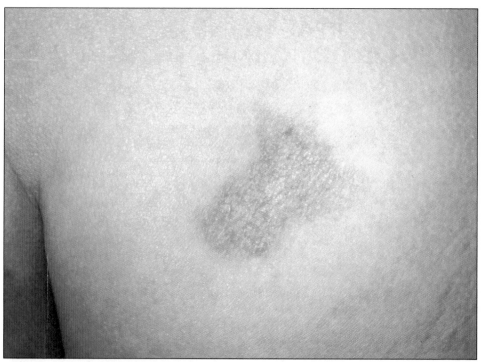

Figure 35. Subcutaneous atrophy after IM keralog injection.

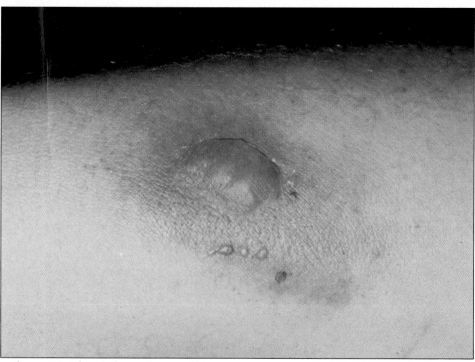

Figure 36. Vincristine extravasation.

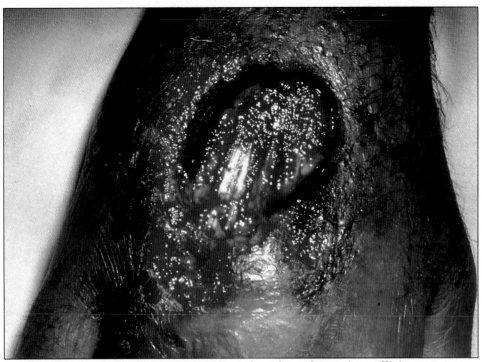

Figure 37. Necrosis after extravasation of methamphetamine. (Illicit use.)

DRUGS OF PARTICULAR INTEREST

PENICILLINS

TABLE 12. TYPES OF ALLERGIC REACTIONS TO PENICILLIN.

Immediate (within 1 hour) and accelerated (1 to 72 hours)

Urticaria
Laryngeal edema
Bronchospasm
Hypotension
Local swelling

Late (after 72 hours)

Morbilliform rash
Serum sickness
Urticaria

Other late reactions

Stevens-Johnson syndrome
Interstitial nephritis
Pulmonary infiltration
Vasculitis
Hemolytic anemia
Neutropenia
Thrombocytopenia

Reproduced with permission from Saxon A, Beall GN, Rohr AS, Adelman DC. Immediate hypersensitivity reactions to beta-lactam antibiotics. *Ann Intern Med.* 1987; 107:204-215.

TABLE 13. UNDERTAKING PENICILLIN ALLERGY SKIN TESTING.

Possible indications

The need to administer penicillin to a person possibly allergic to penicillin.

There is no suitable alternative antibiotic.

The alternatives are: not bactericidal, more costly, difficult to administer, toxic, or requires hospitalization.

To diagnose a recent penicillin allergic reaction.

Not indicated

To document a history of penicillin allergy.

To obtain information for an indefinite time in the future.

For non-IgE-mediated allergic reactions.

Cautions

The information must be used within 72 hours.

Skin testing must be repeated if penicillin is used again.

The test antigens are theoretically capable of sensitizing the patient.

Skin testing can cause reactions; fatalities have resulted from improper testing.

Reproduced with permission from Saxon, et al. Immediate hypersensitivity reactions to beta-lactam antibiotics. *Ann Intern Med.* 1987; 107:204-215.

ADDITIONAL POINTS

1) Only the penicilloyl metabolite, the "major determinant," accounting for 95% of protein-bound drug metabolites, is commercially available.

2) The minor determinants are unstable and not yet commercially available. However physicians at many academic centers synthesize them.

3) Testing with the major determinant alone has a sensitivity of only 76% vs 93% with the major determinant and one minor determinant, benzylpenicillin. Properly performed, testing using major and all minor determinants, with controls, has a sensitivity of >99%—fewer than 1% of patients with negative tests will have a subsequent IgE-mediated skin reaction.

4) The use of "old" aqueous penicillin for testing, in the hope that hydrolysis products will detect allergy to minor determinants, is unacceptable.

5) If minor determinants are not available in one's community or at a nearby academic center, and testing with available determinants is negative, penicillin should be administered with exteme caution in the absence of a clearcut history of urticaria/angioedema/anaphylaxis to penicillin. With such a history, penicillin should not be administered or the patient should be desensitized.

NONSTEROIDAL ANTIINFLAMMATORY DRUGS

Chemical Classification	Generic Name	Brand Name
Salicylates	Acetylate	
	Aspirin	Various
	Nonacetylated	
	Diflunisal	Dolobid
	Salsalate	Disalcid
	Choline magnesium trisalicylate	Trilisate
Acetic acids	Indomethacin	Indocin
	Sulindac	Clinoril
	Tolmetin	Tolectin
	Diclofenac	Voltaren
	Ketorolac	Torodol
	Etodolac	Lodine
Propionic acids	Ibuprofen	Motrin, Advil, Rufen,Nuprin
	Naproxen	Naprosyn
	Fenoprofen	Nalfon
	Ketoprofen	Orudis
	Suprofen	Suprol
	Flurbiprofen	Ansaid
	Nabumetone	Relafen
Anthranilic acids	Mefenamate	Ponstel
	Meclofenamate sodium	Meclomen
Pyrazolones	Phenylbutazone	Azolid, Butazolidin
	Oxyphenbutazone	Oxalid, Tandearil
Oxicams	Piroxicam	Feldene

Modified and reprinted with permission from Roth DE, Spencer LV, Ahrens EM. *Med Clin North Am.* 1989; 73:1275-1298.

MEDICATIONS USED TO TREAT HIV-RELATED DISEASES

CIPROFLOXACIN

Exanthem, pruritis, urticaria, photosensitivity, flushing, angioedema, cutaneous candidiasis, hyperpigmentation, erythema nodosum, erythema multiforme minor, TEN, vasculitis, purpura, vesicles, hyperhidrosis, erythroderma, anaphylactoid reaction, anaphylaxis, acneiform eruption.

COMPOUND Q

"Rash," anaphylaxis.

DDC (DIDEOXYCYTIDINE)

Maculopapular eruption on day 10 or 11 of therapy, erythroderma, papulovesicular lesions, nail changes, angioedema, erythroderma, vesicular or bullous eruption, aphthous stomatitis, lesions on soft palate, tongue and pharynx.

DIDANOSINE (DDI)

Exanthem, pruritus, hyperhidrosis, xerostomia, eczematous eruption, flushing, erythema multiforme major (Stevens-Johnson syndrome); in children as for adults plus impetigo, excoriation and erythema.

ENOXACIN

Photosensitivity, urticaria, exanthem, dermatitis.

FANSIDAR

Erythema multiforme major (Stevens-Johnson syndrome), erythroderma, exanthem, photosensitivity, oral lichenoid eruption, TEN.

FLUCONAZOLE

Exanthem, erythema multiforme major (Stevens-Johnson syndrome {patients were taking other medications, however}), anaphylaxis, pruritus, purpura.

FOSCARNET

Genital and oral ulcerations, fixed drug eruption, phlebitis at infusion site.

ITRACONAZOLE

Exanthem, pruritus, xerostomia, conjunctivitis, edema.

KETOCONAZOLE

Urticaria, anaphylaxis, dermatitis, exfoliative dermatitis, pruritis, alopecia, abnormal hair texture, scalp pustules, xerosis, fixed drug eruption, photodermatitis, exanthem, hyperpigmentation.

OFLOXACIN

Diaphoresis, vasculitis, photosensitivity, angioedema, erythema, pruritus, exanthem, anaphylaxis, urticaria.

PENTAMIDINE (IV)

Exanthem, erythroderma, sterile abscess at injection site, erythema multiforme major (Stevens-Johnson syndrome), gingivitis, oral ulcer, vasculitis, pruritus, urticaria. Morbilliform rashes, erythema, xerosis, desquamation, blepharitis, and urticaria have also occurred with use of inhaled aerosolized pentamidine.

QUINOLONES/RIFAMPIN

These drugs can cause an anaphylactoid reaction, with generalized erythema, edema, and hypotension. This has occurred in patients taking ciprofloxacin on their second course. Drug fever occurring on the first course may be predictive. (Other reactions are listed on p. 151.)

Trimethoprim + Sulfamethoxazole

Exanthem, pruritus, urticaria, dermatitis, erythema multiforme minor, erythema multiforme major (Stevens-Johnson syndrome), vesicular or bullous eruption, TEN, vasculitis, oral mucous membrane lesions including glossitis and erosions, purpura, photosensitivity, pustular reaction, pustular toxic erythema, lupus erythematosus, angioedema, exfoliative dermatitis, Henoch-Schoenlein purpura, serum sickness, conjunctival and sceral injection, periarteritis nodosa-like syndrome, fixed drug eruption.

Zidovudine (AZT)

Exanthem, acne, pruritus, urticaria, brown, blackish or bluish nail discoloration in a diffuse or striate pattern, bluish lunulae, vasculitis, bullous lesions, hyperpigmentation, porphyria cutanea tarda, acneiform eruption, eyelash hypertrichosis, erythema multiforme major (Stevens-Johnson syndrome), mucosal hypermelanosis, oral ulcers.

CANCER CHEMOTHERAPEUTIC AGENTS

ALKYLATING AGENTS

BUSULFAN

Exanthem, urticaria, erythema multiforme minor, purpura, vasculitis, erythema nodosum, oral mucous membrane lesions, alopecia, induction of porphyria cutanea tarda, excessive dryness and fragility of skin, lupus erythematosus, macular erythema, anhidrosis, cheilitis, angioedema, generalized (Addisonian) hyperpigmentation of skin (on neck, upper trunk, nipples, abdomen, palmar creases and on mucous membranes).

CHLORAMBUCIL

Exanthem, pruritus, urticaria, angioedema, exfoliative or eczematous dermatitis, TEN, oral mucous membrane lesions, alopecia, herpes zoster, erythema multiforme minor, pellagra-like eruption.

CYCLOPHOSPHAMIDE

Exanthem, urticaria, dermatitis, erythema multiforme minor, vesicular or bullous eruption, TEN, purpura, lichenoid eruption, acneiform eruption, alopecia, photosensitivity, increased viral and fungal infections, stomatitis, angioedema, anaphylaxis, vasculitis, benign and malignant skin tumors including dermatofibromas, miliaria-like eruption, palmar-plantar erythrodysesthesia syndrome, pruritus, hyperpigmentation of skin, nails, teeth and mucous membranes, nail ridging.

MELPHALAN

Exanthem, vasculitis, oral mucous membrane lesions, alopecia, angioedema, anaphylaxis, hypermelanosis of nails, urticaria, pruritus.

THIOTEPA

Exanthem, pruritus, urticaria, angioedema, purpura, oral mucous membrane lesions, depigmentation, alopecia, hyperpigmentation under occluded skin, redness and burning, bullae, mild erythema.

TOPICAL NITROGEN MUSTARD (MECHLORETHAMINE)

Erythema multiforme minor, squamous cell carcinoma, bullae, purpura, alopecia, exanthem, telangiectasia, immediate hypersensitivity reaction, contact dermatitis, hyperpigmentation with topical use.

Antimetabolites

Azathioprine

Exanthem, urticaria, purpura, alopecia, red discoloration of lunulae, xerostomia, stomatitis, acneiform eruption, photosensitivity, cutaneous neoplasms, erythema multiforme minor, photodistributed hypermelanosis, Raynaud's phenomenon, vasculitis, more frequent cutaneous infections.

Cytarabine

Exanthem, dermatitis, purpura, oral mucous membrane lesions, depigmentation, skin ulceration, freckling, alopecia, angioedema, pruritus, urticaria, palmar-plantar erythrodysesthesia, neutrophilic eccrine hidradenitis, syndrome of fever, malaise, arthralgias, conjunctivitis and maculopapular rash in 24 hours preventable with corticosteroids.

5-Fluorouracil

Exanthem, pruritus, angioedema, dermatitis, vesicular or bullous eruption, lichenoid eruption, alopecia, telangiectasia, scarring, xerosis, fissuring, palmar-plantar erythrodysesthesia, photosensitivity, TEN, bullous pemphigoid, serpentine (postinflammatory) hyperpigmentation along injected veins, isolated blisters or bullous eruption, hypermelanosis in photodistribution, pigmented macules, stomatitis, hyperpigmentation of nails, inflammation of actinic keratoses.

Mercaptopurine

Exanthem, dermatitis, TEN, lupus erythematosus, oral mucous membrane lesions, hyperpigmentation, photosensitivity, pellagra-like eruption, lichenoid eruption, alopecia.

Methotrexate

Exanthem, pruritus, urticaria, eczematous dermatitis, TEN, purpura, vasculitis, photosensitivity, acneiform eruption, depigmentation, hyperpigmentation, ecchymoses, telangiectasia, acne, various cutaneous infections, discoloration of nails, induction of porphyria cutanea tarda, erythema multiforme minor, stomatitis, alopecia, angioedema, exfoliative erythroderma, squamous cell carcinoma, epidermal necrosis and cutaneous ulcers, vesiculation and ulceration over pressure areas, anaphylactoid reaction, Raynaud's phenomenon, paronychia, reactivation of radiation dermatitis and sunburn, palmar-plantar erythrodysesthesia.

Antibiotics

Bleomycin

Exanthem, pruritus, angioedema, eczematous dermatitis, purpura, depigmentation, hyperkeratosis of palms, lichenoid eruption, scleroderma-like fibrosis, alopecia, gray hair, brown discoloration of nails, acrocyanosis, lupus erythematosus, contact dermatitis, hyperpigmented striae, streaky flagellate erythema followed by flagellate hypermelanosis, xerosis, neutrophilic eccrine hydradenitis, stomatitis, oral ulcerations, onycholysis and other nail dystrophy, Raynaud's phenomenon (patients were also on vinblastine), transient penile calcification, inflammatory nodules on the elbows, hands, knees, buttocks.

Dactinomycin

Exanthem, papular-pustular acneiform eruption, alopecia, erythema, hyperpigmentation, exfoliative dermatitis, dermatitis, erythema multiforme minor, TEN, oral mucous membrane lesions, radiation recall. At infusion site: pain, redness, swelling, chemical cellulitis.

Daunorubicin

Exanthem, urticaria, angioedema, oral mucous membrane lesions, reversible alopecia, brown to black nail bands, pain, redness, swelling at infusion site or distally, hypermelanosis.

Doxorubicin

Exanthem, urticaria, dermatitis, vesicular or bullous eruption, purpura, reversible alopecia, necrosis after injection, onycholysis, flushing, erythema, stomatitis, hyperpigmentation of skin, hypermelanosis of nails, radiation recall, chemical cellulitis and phlebitis, urticarial flare proximal to injection site, inflammation of actinic keratoses, palmar-plantar erythrodysesthesia syndrome.

Mithramycin

Exanthem, TEN, purpura, oral mucous membrane lesions; facial erythema and edema followed by desquamation and hyperpigmentation (an early indication of systemic toxicity).

Mitomycin C

Exanthem, pruritus, angioedema, dermatitis, purpura, stomatitis, alopecia, necrosis/sloughing if drug is extravasated during injection, erythema, contact allergic dermatitis, urticaria, vesicular eruption with pruritus.

Plant Alkyloids

Vinblastine

Dermatitis, vesicular or bullous eruption, oral mucous membrane lesions, acneiform eruption, alopecia, skin vesiculation, Raynaud's phenomenon, photosensitivity, isolated blisters or bullous eruption; intralesional injection results in pain, redness, swelling with necrosis of injected lesions at 36-48 hrs.

Vincristine

Exanthem, pruritus, oral mucous membrane lesions, edema, alopecia; pain, redness, swelling at injection site.

Nitrosoureas

BCNU (systemic)

Exanthem, purpura, oral mucous membrane lesions, burning, hyperpigmentation (rare), flushing, conjunctivitis, alopecia.

BCNU (topical)

Hyperpigmentation, irritation, telangiectasia.

CCNU (Lomustine)

Purpura, oral mucous membrane lesions, alopecia, exanthem.

Miscellaneous

Asparaginase

Exanthem, hypersensitivity reactions including urticaria, serum sickness, angioedema and anaphylaxis; purpura, oral mucous membrane lesions, TEN, alopecia.

Cisplatin

Angioedema, purpura, alopecia, oral mucous membrane lesions, "hypersensitivity reactions" that include "anxiety, flushing, burning, tingling, pruritus, cough, dyspnea, diaphoresis, periorbital edema, bronchospasm, vomiting, erythema, urticaria, exanthem, and hypotension" (Weiss RB and Bruno S, *Ann Intern Med* 1981).

Dacarbazine (DTIC®)

Photosensitivity, exanthem, urticaria, angioedema, fixed drug eruption, hypermelanosis of nails, inflammation of actinic keratoses, flushing, anaphylaxis, localized infusion site reactions.

Etoposide

Exanthem, pruritus, oral mucous membrane lesions, reversible alopecia, scaling, anaphylaxis, xerosis, radiation recall, erythema multiforme major (Stevens-Johnson syndrome), acne.

Hydroxyurea

Exanthem, pruritus, fixed drug eruption, dermatitis, erythema multiforme minor, vasculitis, oral mucous membrane lesions, lichenoid eruption, hypermelanosis, facial edema, brown discoloration of nails and rare pigmented longitudinal nail bands, dermatomyositis-like syndrome, alopecia, skin and subcutaneous atrophy, skin ulcerations, skin cancers in photoexposed areas.

Interferons

Exanthem, pruritus, alopecia, purpura, hypertrichosis, increased growth of eyelashes, systemic sclerosis, bleeding gums or sore gums, xerostomia, edema, xerosis, cyanosis, flushing of the skin, Raynaud's phenomenon, urticaria, exacerbation or induction of psoriasis or herpes, acne, fungal infection, eczematous eruption, telangiectasia, photosensitivity, erythema/transient urticaria at injection site, hyperhidrosis.

INTERLEUKIN 2

Local reaction at injection site, erythroderma with necrotic lesions and purpura or tense blisters, mucositis, glossitis, punctate superficial ulcers, erosions in scars, erythrodermic flares of psoriasis, icterus, erythema nodosum, basal cell cancer and other tumors at injection site, alopecia, macular erythema with burning and pruritus on head, neck and chest, pemphigus, erythema nodosum, exanthem, petechiae on legs, facial/palmar-plantar edema, urticarial papules, urticaria; cutaneous toxicity in 96% of patients and 72% of cycles within 36-72h—recurrences may be earlier but milder on subsequent cycles.

PROCARBAZINE

Exanthem, pruritus, urticaria, angioedema, dermatitis, TEN, purpura, oral mucous membrane lesions, herpes, dermatitis, alopecia, hyperpigmentation, photosensitivity, flushing "Antabuse-like" effect.

THIOGUANINE

Oral mucous membrane lesions, exanthem, photosensitivity, alopecia.

FUTURE DIRECTIONS

How can we understand the mechanisms that cause many drug reactions?

How can we predict which patients are at risk for adverse cutaneous reactions?

The studies noted below have investigated the metabolism and detoxification of drugs, and point to our future understanding of mechanisms and risk factors for adverse cutaneous drug reactions.

1. DILANTIN HYPERSENSITIVITY AND ARENE OXIDE METABOLITES

Toxic arene oxide metabolites of phenytoin are made by hepatic cytochrome P-450 enzymes and are detoxified by a variety of enzymes, including epoxide hydrolase. Compared with control cells, the lymphocytes of several patients with dilantin hypersensitivity demonstrated increased toxicity from these metabolites, and resembled control cells whose epoxide hydrolase was inhibited.

Shear NH, Spielberg SP. The anticonvulsant hypersensitivity syndrome: *In-vitro* assessment of risk. *J Clin Invest.* 1988; 82:1826-1832.

Spielberg SP, Gordon GB, Blake DA, et al. Predisposition to phenytoin hepatotoxicity assessed *In-vitro*. *N Engl J Med.* 1981; 305:722-727.

2. SULFONAMIDE HYPERSENSITIVITY AND ACETYLATION STATUS

Patients with sulfonamide hypersensitivity reactions were found to be slow acetylators, and their lymphocytes were much more sensitive to hydroxylamine metabolites of sulfas than controls.

Rieder, Uetrecht J, Shear NH, et al. Diagnosis of sulfonamide hypersensitivity reactions by *In-vitro* "rechallenge" with hydroxylamine metabolites. *Ann Intern Med.* 1989; 110:286-289.

Shear NH, Spielberg SP, Grant DM, Tang BK. Differences in metabolism of sulfonamides predisposing to idiosyncratic toxicity. *Ann Intern Med.* 1986; 105:179-184.

3. ACETAMINOPHEN TOXICITY AND GLUTATHIONE SYNTHETASE DEFICIENCY

Microsomal enzyme-generated metabolites of acetaminophen are detoxified by conjugation with glutathione. Lymphocytes from a patient with glutathione synthetase deficiency and with lower levels of glutathione were much more sensitive to these toxic metabolites than control lymphocytes.

Spielberg SP, Gordon GB. Glutathione synthetase-deficient lymphocytes and acetaminophen toxicity. *Clin Pharmacol Ther.* 1981; 29:51-55.

4. PROTEIN C LEVELS AND COUMARIN NECROSIS

Many patients with coumarin necrosis have decreased levels of protein C, a vitamin K-dependent anticoagulant protease zymogen. Coumarin lowers protein C and Factor VII levels before Factors IX and X and prothrombin, causing a transient hypercoagulable state, promoting necrosis in the skin.

Broekmans AW, Bertina RM, Loelinger EA, et al. Protein C and the development of skin necrosis during anticoagulant therapy (letter). *Thromb Haemost.* 1983; 49:251.

Rose VL, Kwann HC, Williamson K, et al. Protein C antigen deficiency and warfarin necrosis. *Am J Clin Phthal.* 1986; 86:653-655.

5. INVESTIGATION OF OXICAM-INDUCED PHOTOSENSITIVITY

Normal subjects and patients with piroxicam photosensitivity were patch and photopatch tested using two known photoproducts of piroxicam as well as UVA pre-irradiated piroxicam itself. Positive patch tests were obtained only in piroxicam-sensitive individuals exposed to pre-irradiated piroxicam. Thus, minor or unidentified photoproducts of piroxicam may be responsible for piroxicam photosensitivity. These conclusions were also suggested by a previous study.

Serrano G, Fortea JM, Latasa JM, et al. Oxicam-induced photosensitivity. Patch and photopatch testing studies with tenoxicam and piroxicam photoproducts in normal subjects and in piroxicam-diroxicam photosensitive patients. *J Am Acad Dermatol.* 1992; 26:545-548.

Kochevar IE, Morison WL, Lamm JL. Possible mechanism of piroxicam-induced photosensitivity. *Arch Dermatol.* 1986; 122:1283-1287.

6. INVESTIGATION OF FAMILIAL HYPERSENSITIVITY REACTIONS TO PHENYTOIN

Three siblings developed a hypersensitivity reaction to phenytoin, consisting of fever, rash, adenopathy, and hepatitis. One patient tolerated phenobarbital. Peripheral blood mononuclear cells from the three patients and five other siblings were incubated with phenytoin, carbamazepine, and phenobarbital metabolites produced by a hepatic microsomal system *in vitro*. All three patients and four of five siblings had increased toxicity to phenytoin and carbamazepine, but not to phenobarbital. The familial propensity toward drug hypersensitivity was thus confirmed *in vitro*.

Gennis MA, Vermuri R, Burns EA, et al. Familial occurrence of hypersensitivity to phenytoin. *Am J Med.* 1991; 91:631-634.

7. *In vitro* Investigation of Sorbinil Hypersensitivity

Sorbinil, a new drug investigated in diabetic neuropathy and retinopathy, produces fever, rash and myalgias in 10% of subjects. The toxicity of *in vitro* generated sorbinil metabolites was assessed. Lymphocytes from controls who tolerated the drug exhibited 7.9% cell death compared with 23.4% of lymphocytes from three patients with a hypersensitivity reaction to sorbinil.

Spielberg SP, Shear NH, Cannon M, et al. *In-vitro* assessment of the hypersensitivity syndrome associated with sorbinil. *Ann Intern Med.* 1991; 114:720.

8. Mechanism of Toxicity of Hydroxylamine Metabolites of Sulfamethoxazole

Hydroxylamine metabolites of sulfamethoxazole appear to be toxic to lymphocytes from patients sensitive to sulfamethoxazole compared to controls. The intracellular targets of these metabolites were investigated in lymphocytes. It was found that early inhibition of intracellular esterase activity correlated with cell death.

Leeder JS, Dosch HM, Spielberg SP, et al. Cellular toxicity of sulfamethoxazole reactive metabolites—I. inhibition of intracellular esterase activity prior to cell death. *Biochem Pharmacol.* 1991; 41:567-74.

9. Cutaneous Reactions Associated with the Clinical Use of Biologic Response Modulators

In addition to the studies cited above, the availability and pharmacologic use of cytokines and other endogenous immunomodulators are providing new insights into skin reactivity. Our present knowledge of the production of cytokines by immune and non-immune cells of the skin and our understanding of the cutaneous effects of cytokines and immunomodulators used pharmacologically, may contribute to future studies of the role of cytokines in adverse cutaneous reactions to other classes of drugs.

Reporting Adverse Reactions

Most physicians recognize that the reporting of adverse drug reactions only begins with approval and marketing. The reasons that premarketing studies fail to fully identify adverse reactions have been reviewed* and include the small size of the premarketing study population, the short duration of pre-marketing studies, the emphasis of phase III studies on efficacy, tight inclusion-exclusion criteria, early discontinuation of medication with onset of adverse reactions, high drop-out rate, and the statistical treatment of adverse reactions. It was pointed out that to detect an adverse reaction with a 1% incidence, more than 300 patients who are at risk must be examined. Also, the drop-outs of a study, who might have idiosyncratic reactions, are often not studied, and may represent patients with unusual genetic predispositions. Therefore, it falls on the shoulders of individual clinicians to recognize and report adverse reactions.

*Naranjo CA, Jones JK (eds). *Idiosyncratic adverse drug reactions: Impact on drug development and clinical use after marketing.* New York, NY: Excerpta Medica; 1990.

Specify

The type of reaction: be as precise as possible in describing the type of skin rash and distribution. The term "rash" is not as helpful as hives, maculopapular eruption, erythema multiforme, etc.

The date of onset of the reaction.

The date of first administration of the suspected medication, dose and route of administration.

All other medications used by the patient and their dates of first administration or readministration if there has been a break in treatment; include topicals where relevant, eye drops, suppositories, etc. Specify the dose and recent changes in the dose.

Medical conditions for which the suspected medication was prescribed.

Other medical problems of the patient.

The response to discontinuation of treatment.

The response to readministration (if performed).

Sequelae.

Adverse drug reactions should be reported to the hospital pharmacy or to the appropriate committee overseeing adverse drug reactions. The problem list in the patients' chart should be updated. In addition, physicians should report the reaction to the manufacturer or directly to the FDA, MEDWATCH, 5600 Fishers Lane, Rockville, MD 20852-9787, or by FAX to 1-800-FDA-0178. Call 1-800-FDA-1088 for information or to request MEDWATCH FDA Form 3500.

References

General

Baker H. Drug Reactions. In: Rook A, Wilkinson DS, Ebling FJG, Champion RH, Burton JL (eds): *Textbook of dermatology*. 4th ed. Boston, MA: Blackwell Scientific Publications, Inc.; 1986, pp 1239-1279.

Bork K. *Cutaneous side effects of drugs*. Philadelphia, PA: W.B. Saunders Co; 1988. (A complete text with photos.)

Breathnach SM, Hintner H. *Adverse drug reactions and the skin*. Oxford, England: Blackwell Scientific Publications; 1992. (A complete text with summaries of clinical syndromes, data on pathomechanisms, and excellent photographs. Organized by reaction type and by drug.)

Bruinsma W (ed): *A guide to drug eruptions*. 5th ed. Amsterdam, Netherlands: Free University Amsterdam; 1990. (Available through the American Overseas Book Co Inc. in Norwood, NJ. No photos but a comprehensive and easy to use handbook with more than 850 references.)

Litt JZ, Pawlak WA, Jr. *Drug eruption reference manual*. Cleveland, OH: Wal-Zac Publishing Co; 1992. (An exceptionally easy to use and exhaustive list of cutaneous reactions each with original journal reference(s) or source. Also available on disk for IBM-PC. Lists more than 280 drugs. Order tel. 216-464-7200, fax 216-464-0020.)

Mehta M (ed). *PDR guide to drug interactions, side effects, indications*. 46th ed. Montvale, NJ: Medical Economics Data; 1992. (Keyed to citations in the *Physician's desk reference*. Individual reactions can be accessed and various drugs causing those reactions are listed.)

Physicians' Desk Reference. 47th ed. Montvale, NJ: Medical Economics Data; 1993.

Zürcher K, Krebs A. *Hautnebenwirkungen interner arzneimittel*. Basel, Switzerland: S. Karger AG; 1980.

Zürcher K, Krebs A. *Cutaneous drug reactions*. Basel, Switzerland: S. Karger AG; 1992. (An excellent reference text of 570 pages with almost 5600 references. Data are listed by drug and also by reaction type. Many details are also given.)

Making a diagnosis

Shear NH. Diagnosing cutaneous adverse reactions to drugs. *Arch Dermatol.* 1990;126:94-97.

Classification

Wintroub BU, Stern R. Cutaneous drug reactions: Pathogenesis and clinical classification. *J Am Acad Dermatol.* 1985;13:167-179.

Urticaria and exanthems (maculopapular rashes)

Arndt KA, Jick H. Rates of cutaneous reactions to drugs. A report from the Boston Collaborative Drug Surveillance Program. *JAMA.* 1976;235:918-923.

Bigby M, Jick S, Jick H, Arndt K. Drug induced cutaneous reactions: A report from the Boston Collaborative Drug Surveillance Program on 13,438 inpatients, 1975-1983. *JAMA.* 1986;256:3358-3363.

Photosensitivity

Epstein JH, Wintroub BU. Photosensitivity due to drugs. *Drugs.* 1985;30:42-57.

FIXED DRUG ERUPTION

Kanwar AJ, Bharija SC, Singh M, Belhaj MS. Ninety-eight fixed drug eruptions with provocation tests. *Dermatologica.* 1988; 177:274-279.

Korkij W, Soltani K. Fixed drug eruption. A brief review. *Arch Dermatol.* 1984; 120:520-524.

Shelley WB, Shelley ED. Nonpigmenting fixed drug eruption as a distinctive reaction pattern: Examples caused by sensitivity to pseudoephedrine hydrochloride and tetrahydrozoline. *J Am Acad Dermatol.* 1987; 17:403-407.

LICHENOID DRUG ERUPTION

Boyd AS, Nelder KH. Lichen planus. *J Am Acad Dermatol.* 1991; 25:593-619.

Halevy S. and Shai A. Lichenoid Drug Eruptions. *J Am Acad Dermatol.* 1993; 24:249-255.

West AJ, Berger TG, Leboit PE. A comparative histopathologic study of photodistributed and non-photodistributed lichenoid drug eruptions. *J Am Acad Dermatol.* 1990; 23:689-693.

TOXIC EPIDERMAL NECROLYSIS

Bastuji-Garin S, Rzany B, Stern RS, Shear NH, Naldi L, Roujeau JC. Clinical classification of cases of toxic epidermal necrolysis, Stevens-Johnson syndrome, and erythema multiforme. *Arch Dermatol.* 1993; 129:92-96.

Goldstein SM, Wintroub BU, Elias PE, Wuepper KD. Toxic epidermal necrolysis: Unmuddying the waters. *Arch Dermatol.* 1987; 123:1153-1156.

Heimbach DM, Engrau LH, Marvin JA, et al. Toxic epidermal necrolysis: A step forward in treatment. *JAMA.* 1987; 257:2171-2175.

Heng MCY, Allen SG. Efficacy of cyclophosphamide in toxic epidermal necrolysis. Clinical and pathophysiologic aspects. *J Am Acad Dermatol.* 1991; 925:778-786.

Roujeau JC, Chosidow O, Saiag P, Guillaume J-C. Toxic epidermal necrolysis (Lyell syndrome). *J Am Acad Dermatol.* 1990; 23: 1039-1058.

ERYTHEMA MULTIFORME

Bastuji-Garin S, Rzany B, Stern RS, Shear NH, Naldi L, Roujeau JC. Clinical classification of cases of toxic epidermal necrolysis, Stevens-Johnson syndrome, and erythema multiforme. *Arch Dermatol.* 1993; 129:92-96.

Huff JC, Weston WL, Tonnesen MG. Erythema multiforme: A critical review of characteristics, diagnostic criteria, and causes. *J Am Acad Dermatol.* 1983; 8:763-775.

Renfro L, Grant-Kels JM, Feder HM, et al. Controversy: are systemic steroids indicated in the treatment of erythema multiforme? *Pediatric Dermatol.* 1989; 6:43-50.

EXFOLIATIVE ERYTHRODERMA

Nicolis GD, Helwig EB. Exfoliative dermatitis: A clinicopathologic study of 135 cases. *Arch Dermatol.* 1973; 108:788-797.

DRUG-INDUCED ALOPECIA

Brodin MB. Drug-induced alopecia. *Dermatol Clin.* 1987; 5:571-579.

DRUG-INDUCED PIGMENTARY CHANGES

Lerner EA, Sober AJ. Chemical and pharmacologic agents that cause hyperpigmentation or hypopigmentation of the skin. *Dermatol Clin.* 1988; 6:327-337.

Steele TE, Ashby J. Desipramine-related slate-gray skin pigmentation (Letter). *J Clin Psychopharmacol.* 1993; 13:76.

CHEMOTHERAPY-ASSOCIATED PALMAR-PLANTAR ERYTHRODYSESTHESIA SYNDROME

Lokich JJ, Moore C. Chemotherapy-associated palmar-plantar dysesthesia syndrome. *Ann Intern Med.* 1984; 101:798-800.

Rongioletti F, Ballestrero A, Bogliolo F, et al. Necrotizing eccrine squamous syringometaplasia presenting as acral erythema. *J Cutan Pathol.* 1991; 18:453-456.

Vukelja SJ, Sharkey MJ, Baker WJ and Berger TC. Pericarditis associated with acral erythema of chemotherapy: A syndrome of cutaneous and mucosal toxicities. *Cutis.* 1993; 52:89-90.

Waltzer JF, Flowers FP. Bullous variant of chemotherapy-induced acral erythema. *Arch Dermatol.* 1993; 129:43-44.

NEUTROPHILIC ECCRINE HIDRADENITIS

Harrist TJ, Fine JD, Berman RS, Murphy GF, Mihm MC. Neutrophilic eccrine hidradenitis. *Arch Dermatol.* 1982; 118:263-266.

Margolis DJ, Gross PR. Neutrophilic eccrine hidradenitis: A case report and review of the literature. *Cutis.* 1991; 48:198-200.

Smith KJ, Skelton HG, et al. Neutrophilic eccrine hidradenitis in HIV-infected patients. *J Am Acad Dermatol.* 1990; 23:945-947.

SYRINGOSQUAMOUS METAPLASIA/ECCRINE SQUAMOUS SYRINGOMETAPLASIA

Bahwan J, Malhotra R. Syringosquamous metaplasia: A distinctive eruption in patients receiving chemotherapy. *Am J Dermatopathol.* 1990; 12:1-6.

Hurt MA, Halvorson RD Petr C Jr, et al. Eccrine squamous syringometaplasia: A cutaneous sweat gland reaction in the histologic spectrum of "chemotherapy-associated eccrine hidradenitis" and neutrophilic eccrine hidradenitis." *Arch Dermatol.* 1990; 126:73-77.

VITAMIN K HYPERSENSITIVITY

Sanders MN, Winkelmann RK. Cutaneous reactions to vitamin K. *J Am Acad Dermatol.* 1988; 19:699-704.

ALLOPURINOL TOXICITY/HYPERSENSITIVITY SYNDROME

Hande KR, Noone RM, Stone WJ, et al. Severe Allopurinol Toxicity. Description and guidelines for prevention in patients with renal insufficiency. *Am J Med.* 1985; 76:47-56.

Lupton GP, Odom RB. The allopurinol hypersensitivity syndrome. *J Am Acad Dermatol.* 1979; 1:365-374.

DRUG-INDUCED LUPUS ERYTHEMATOSUS

Cush JJ, Goldings EA. Drug induced lupus: clinical spectrum and pathogenesis. *Am J Med Sci.* 1985; 290:36-44, C3.

Uetrecht J. Drug metabolism by leukocytes and its role in drug-induced lupus and other idiosyncratic drug reactions. *Critical Rev Toxicol.* 1990; 20:213-235.

CUTANEOUS ERUPTION OF LYMPHOCYTE RECOVERY

Bauer DJ, Hood AF, Horn TD. Histologic comparison of autologous graft-vs-host reaction and cutaneous eruption of lymphocyte recovery. *Arch Dermatol.* 1993; 129:855-858.

Horn TD, Redd JV, Karp JE et al. Cutaneous eruptions of lymphocyte recovery. *Arch Dermatol.* 1989; 125:1512-1517.

PENICILLIN REACTIONS

Adelman D. Penicillin allergy. *Western J Med.* 1991; 154,456.

Saxon A, Beall GN, Rohr AS, Adelman DC. Immediate hypersensitivity reactions to beta-lactam antibiotics. *Ann Intern Med.* 1987; 107:204-215.

NONSTEROIDAL ANTIINFLAMMATORY DRUGS

Roth DE, Spencer LV, Ahrens EM. Cutaneous reactions to drugs used for rheumatologic disorders. *Med Clin North Am.* 1989; 73:1275-1298.

Stern Rs, Bigby M. An expanded profile of cutaneous reactions to non-steroidal anti-inflammatory drugs. *JAMA.* 1984; 252:1433-1437.

CHEMOTHERAPY-ASSOCIATED ERUPTIONS (see p 101)

General

Fitzpatrick JE. The cutaneous histopathology of chemotherapeutic reactions. *J Cutan Pathol.* 1993; 20:1-14.

Cisplatin

Weiss RB and Bruno S. Hypersensitivity reactions to cancer chemotherapeutic agents. *Ann Intern Med.* 1981; 94:66-72.

Hydroxyurea

Richard M, Truchetet F, Friedel J, et al. Skin lesions simulating chronic dermatomyositis during long-term hydroxyurea therapy. *J Am Acad Dermatol.* 1989; 21:797-799.

Interleukin 2

Wolkenstein P, Chosidow O, Wechsler J, et al. Cutaneous side effects associated with interleukin 2 administration for metastatic melanoma. *J Am Acad Dermatol.* 1993; 28:66-70.

CALCIUM CHANNEL BLOCKERS

Stern R, Khalsa JH. Cutaneous adverse reactions associated with calcium channel blockers. *Arch Intern Med.* 1989; 149:829-832

ACKNOWLEDGMENTS

We thank the following individuals for their contributions:

Linda Beets-Shay, MD; Fig. 19
Timothy G. Berger, MD; Figs. 6, 8, 10, 28-30, 36
Axel Hoke, MD; Figs. 35 and 37
Jorge Kershenovich, MD; Fig. 11
Marketa Limova, MD; Fig. 12
David J. Margolis, MD and Paul R. Gross, MD; Fig. 32
Richard B. Odom, MD; Fig. 2
Vera H. Price, MD; Fig. 27
John R. T. Reeves, MD; Figs. 1, 34
Steven Shpall, MD; Figs. 17, 23-26, 31

Figures 15 and 16 are courtesy of the Department of Dermatology, University of California, San Francisco, and Figure 22 is courtesy of the Department of Dermatology, Harvard Medical School.

We are grateful to Daniel Adelman, MD, Kerry L. Blacker, MD, Timothy G. Berger, MD, John H. Epstein, MD, Timothy H. McCalmont, MD, Vera H. Price, MD, Robert S. Stern, MD, and Herschel S. Zackheim, MD, for their advice and comments, and to Anne Maczulak, PhD, for her research.

INDIVIDUAL DRUGS AND REPORTED ADVERSE CUTANEOUS REACTIONS

INTRODUCTION

PROBLEMS IN COMPILING A LIST OF ADVERSE REACTIONS ASSOCIATED WITH DRUGS

We have attempted in the following section to present many of the cutaneous reactions reported for individual drugs. There is probably no single, complete listing of adverse cutaneous reactions to drugs. All the sources that we examined were in agreement on many of the reactions, but often a particular reaction or multiple reactions appeared in one reference and not in another. This is probably due to the lack of any single resource, institution, or journal to which all reports of drug reactions are submitted. Reports must, therefore, be compiled from the medical literature, using both English and non-English journals, and from pharmaceutical companies. Computer searches for cutaneous reactions are often not efficient because reports of therapeutic studies that mention adverse reactions rarely list "adverse reaction" or "rash" as a keyword. Several authors now are attempting to compile complete and updated records using multiple sources. The availability of computer technology may facilitate this process. Clinicians should probably never rule out the possibility of a drug causing a particular reaction because that reaction fails to appear in this handbook or in another reference. Conversely, it is not unlikely that some reports may have incorrectly attributed particular reactions to a specific medication.

DIFFICULTIES IN USING COMPENDIA OF DRUG REACTIONS

As discussed and illustrated by the several Boston Collaborative Drug Surveillance Program reports (see p. 9), it is important that we know the statistical chance of a particular drug causing a particular eruption. However, our knowledge and such data are often incomplete, and the more common types of adverse cutaneous reactions may be caused by many drugs. Therefore, the medical history and the response to dechallenge are critical in identifying the offending drug. Many of the listings that follow are based on single reports, and therefore probably reflect rare events. Thus, we need to make the distinction between reports that help us to explain the dermatologic problem of a single patient from reports that influence our choice of medications. For example, there are several drugs that seem to be likely to exacerbate psoriasis, and it may be wise to avoid use of these drugs in a particular patient. However, exacerbation of psoriasis, or psoriasiform rash have been reported for many more drugs. Finally, the details of each report cannot be presented in this handbook or in most texts. Therefore, clinicians will need to consult the original reference in unusual cases for details concerning description of morphology, response to treatment, duration, morbidity, etc. Referring to original articles will also allow practitioners to specifically evaluate the validity of each report. Several of the texts listed on p. 106 do an excellent job of providing such references, and are highly recommended.

DIFFICULTIES IN BEDSIDE DIAGNOSIS

Many critically ill patients receive multiple therapeutic interventions and multiple drugs. In addition, many new drugs, including cancer chemotherapeutic agents, and biologic response modifiers cause many reactions that do not fall neatly into classic morphologic categories. Some reactions seem to occur primarily in patients treated with particular combination regimens. The careful, systematic and prospective study of many patients on similar, although complex, regimens will be needed to shed further light on cutaneous responses to such agents.

Notes

Reactions that appear to occur most "commonly" with each drug (in > 1% of patients) are italicized.

Cutaneous eruptions are sometimes incompletely or inadequately described and documented. Hence, there is some ambiguity regarding certain reactions.

1) "Dermatitis" refers to seborrheic, eczematous or exfoliative dermatitis. At times only "dermatitis" is listed as a cutaneous reaction in primary sources and reports without further description. Examination of primary sources is recommended for further details of individual reactions.

2) "Vesicular or bullous eruption" refers to reports of vesicles, isolated bullae, or widespread bullae. This may include pemphigoid-like or pemphigus-like reactions as noted.

3) "Vasculitis" in some texts appears to refer to reports that describe palpable purpura or purpuric eruptions often on the lower legs, that are not associated with thrombocytopenia. While these clinical reports may suggest leukocytoclastic vasculitis, the clinical-pathologic correlation in many reports is absent or incomplete. For example, the documentation of vasculitis caused by prednisone or prednisolone seems to be poor. We list those drugs for which reports of vasculitis appear suggestive of true leukocytoclastic vasculitis as this entity is currently understood.

4) "Lupus erythematosus" refers either to induction, aggravation of systemic lupus erythematosus, discoid lupus erythematosus, or to a positive ANA. See pp. 78-81 for further details.

5) "Purpura" refers to either thrombocytopenic purpura or "purpura" not otherwise described.

LISTING OF ADVERSE CUTANEOUS REACTIONS BY DRUG

Acetaminophen
exanthem, pruritus, urticaria, angioedema, fixed drug eruption, dermatitis, purpura, erythema nodosum, alopecia, erythema multiforme minor, erythroderma, anaphylactoid reaction

Acetazolamide
exanthem, pruritus, urticaria, erythema multiforme minor, vesicular or bullous eruption, TEN, lupus erythematosus, lichenoid eruption, hirsutism, "tingling" feeling in extremities, purpura, isolated blisters or bullous eruption

ACTH (adrenocorticotropic hormone)
changes of skin color - *generalized brown,* hypertrichosis, hirsutism, *acneiform eruption,* angioedema, erythema multiforme minor, striae, hyperpigmentation of nails, oral mucous membrane lesions, discoloration of oral mucosa, purpura, exanthem, vasculitis, papules

Acyclovir
edema, *exanthem,* alopecia, pruritus, *urticaria,* eczematous eruption, lichenoid eruption

Adriamycin - see Doxorubicin

Albumin: Human
exanthem, urticaria

Alcuronium
exanthem

Aldesleukin - see Interleukin 2

Allopurinol
exanthem, pruritus, urticaria, angioedema, dermatitis, erythema multiforme minor, erythema multiforme major (Stevens-Johnson syndrome), TEN, vasculitis, oral mucous membrane lesions, alopecia, fixed drug eruption, exfoliative dermatitis, lupus erythematosus, purpura, erythematous papules and plaques, acneiform eruption, ichthyosiform dermatitis, lichen planus, lymphocytoma cutis, onycholysis, polyarteritis nodosa-like syndrome

Amantadine
exanthem, pruritus, hypertrichosis, xerostomia, *livedo reticularis,* photosensitivity, *peripheral edema, alopecia*

Amikacin
exanthem, pruritus, dermatitis

Amiloride

exanthem, pruritus, xerostomia, alopecia, purpura

Aminocaproic acid

exanthem, pruritus

Aminoglutethimide

exanthem, pruritus, urticaria, angioedema, oral mucous membrane lesions, lupus erythematosus, pustular psoriasis-like eruption, exfoliative dermatitis, anaphylactoid reaction

Aminophylline

pruritus, urticaria, dermatitis, lupus erythematosus, alopecia, exfoliative dermatitis

Amiodarone

exanthem, *pruritus, urticaria,* erythema nodosum, photodermatitis, *bluish or slate-gray changes in skin color in light exposed area, photosensitivity,* erythema, alopecia, hyperhidrosis, vasculitis, flushing, iododerma, hypertrichosis, exacerbation of psoriasis, exfoliative dermatitis, *purpura*

Amitriptyline

exanthem, pruritus, urticaria, angioedema, dermatitis, vesicular or bullous eruption, purpura, vasculitis, oral mucous membrane lesions including xerostomia, photosensitivity, hyperhidrosis, exfoliative dermatitis, alopecia

Amoxicillin

exanthem, urticaria, oral mucous membrane lesions including xerostomia, pustular eruption, erythema multiforme minor, erythema multiforme major (Stevens-Johnson syndrome), exfoliative dermatitis, fixed drug eruption, anaphylaxis

Amphetamine

exanthem, urticaria, fixed drug eruption, dermatitis, vesicular or bullous eruption, purpura, vasculitis, alopecia, acneiform eruption, xerostomia

Amphotericin B

exanthem, pruritus, purpura, generalized erythema, anaphylactoid reaction, flushing

Ampicillin

exanthem, pruritus, *urticaria,* angioedema, fixed drug eruption, dermatitis, erythema multiforme minor, erythema multiforme major (Stevens-Johnson syndrome), vesicular or bullous eruption, TEN, purpura, vasculitis, lupus erythematosus, *oral mucous membrane lesions* including black hairy tongue, exfoliative dermatitis, pustular exanthem, anaphylaxis

Antimony

exanthem, pruritus, urticaria, angioedema, fixed drug eruption, dermatitis, purpura

Antipyrine

exanthem, pruritus, urticaria, *fixed drug eruption,* erythema multiforme minor, vesicular or bullous eruption, TEN, purpura, erythema nodosum, lupus erythematosus, oral mucous membrane lesions

Antithymocyte globulin

pruritus, *urticaria, purpura,* wheals at injection site, alopecia, *exanthem, palmar-plantar erythema,* vasculitis

Aprobarbital

exanthem, purpura, fixed drug eruption

Arsenic

exanthem, pruritus, urticaria, *angioedema,* fixed drug eruption, dermatitis, erythema multiforme minor, vesicular or bullous eruption, purpura, vasculitis, erythema nodosum, lupus erythematosus, *oral mucous membrane lesions,* lichenoid eruption, changes of skin color - hypermelanosis or depigmentation, alopecia, *cutaneous tumors,* keratoses, photosensitivity, exfoliative dermatitis, exacerbation of porphyria cutanea tarda, *palmar-plantar keratoderma, palmar hyperhidrosis*

Asparaginase

exanthem, hypersensitivity reactions including urticaria, serum sickness, angioedema and anaphylaxis; purpura, *oral mucous membrane lesions,* TEN, alopecia

Aspirin

exanthem, alopecia, pemphigus, TEN, erythema nodosum, *pruritus,* hyperhidrosis, *urticaria,* lupus erythematosus, vasculitis, exfoliative dermatitis, fixed drug eruption, isolated blisters or bullous eruption, lichenoid eruption, oral ulceration, angioedema, erythema multiforme minor, erythema multiforme major (Stevens-Johnson syndrome), purpura, pustular psoriasis, anaphylactoid reaction

Astemizole

exanthem, angioedema, edema, photosensitivity, pruritus, dermatitis

Atenolol

exanthem, dry eyes, psoriasiform eruption, pustular psoriasis, lichen planus-like eruption, anaphylaxis, alopecia, vitiligo, acrocyanosis, peripheral skin necrosis, pseudolymphoma

Atropine

exanthem, pruritus, urticaria, fixed drug eruption, dermatitis, erythema multiforme minor, erythema multiforme major (Stevens-Johnson syndrome), vesicular or bullous eruption, purpura, vasculitis, oral mucous membrane lesions, xerostomia, flushing, exfoliative dermatitis

Aurofin - see Gold

Aurothioglucose - see Gold

Azatadine
urticaria, photosensitivity, xerostomia, exanthem

Azathioprine
exanthem, urticaria, purpura, *alopecia, red discoloration of lunulae,* xerostomia, stomatitis, acneiform eruption, photosensitivity, *cutaneous neoplasms,* erythema multiforme minor, *photodistributed hypermelanosis,* Raynaud's phenomenon, vasculitis, *more frequent cutaneous infections*

AZT - see Zidovudine

Aztreonam
exanthem, pruritus, purpura, erythema multiforme minor, urticaria, angioedema, hyperhidrosis, exfoliative dermatitis, petechiae, flushing, diaphoresis

Bacampicillin
exanthem, urticaria, erythema multiforme minor, exfoliative dermatitis

Baclofen
urticaria, exanthem, *pruritus,* ankle edema, hyperhidrosis

BCG (Bacille Calmette-Guerin)
hypersensitivity, bullous eruption, TEN, erythema multiforme minor, erythema nodosum, vasculitis, exanthem, pruritus, vesicular or bullous eruption, urticaria, dermatitis, purpura, lupus erythematosus, disseminated tuberculosis

BCNU (Carmustine)
exanthem, purpura, oral mucous membrane lesions, burning, hyperpigmentation (rare), flushing, conjunctivitis, alopecia after systemic use. Hyperpigmentation, irritation, telangiectasia after topical use.

Benactyzine
exanthem, xerostomia

Benzathine penicillin
erythema multiforme minor, exanthem, exfoliative dermatitis, urticaria, TEN, erythema nodosum, pruritus, isolated blisters or bullous eruption

Benzocaine
exanthem, urticaria, dermatitis (contact allergy), burning, stinging, pruritus, erythema, edema

Benzoic acid
urticaria, vasculitis

Benztropine
exanthem, xerostomia

Bepridil
exanthem, hyperhidrosis

Beta carotene
dermatitis, orange-yellow coloration of skin

Bethanechol
vesicular or bullous eruption, lupus erythematosus, flushing, hyperhidrosis

Biperiden
exanthem, pruritus, xerostomia

Bisacodyl
fixed drug eruption

Bismuth
exanthem, pruritus, urticaria, fixed drug eruption, dermatitis, erythema multiforme minor, vesicular or bullous eruption, vasculitis, lupus erythematosus, stomatitis, lichenoid eruption, gray-blue changes of color of skin and gingival mucosa, alopecia, photosensitivity

Bleomycin
exanthem, pruritus, angioedema, *eczematous dermatitis,* purpura, depigmentation, hyperkeratosis of palms, lichenoid eruption, scleroderma-like fibrosis, *alopecia,* gray hair, brown discoloration of nails, acrocyanosis, lupus erythematosus, contact dermatitis, hyperpigmented striae, streaky flagellate erythema followed by *flagellate hypermelanosis,* xerosis, neutrophilic eccrine hydradenitis, *stomatitis, oral ulcerations,* onycholysis and other *nail dystrophy,* Raynaud's phenomenon (patients were also on vinblastine), transient penile calcification, inflammatory nodules on the elbows, hands, knees, buttocks

Borate
exanthem, erythema multiforme minor, alopecia

Boric acid
alopecia

Bretylium
exanthem, flushing, hyperhidrosis

Bromine
changes of skin color—blotchy hypermelanosis, acneiform eruption, bromoderma, fixed drug eruption, erythema multiforme minor, erythema nodosum, isolated blisters or bullous eruption

Bromocriptine

exanthem, vasculitis, alopecia, xerostomia, hyperhidrosis, flushing, erythromelalgia, livedo reticularis, purpura, morphea-like lesions, anaphylaxis, reversible blanching of fingers

Bumetanide

exanthem, erythema multiforme minor, purpura, pseudoporphyria, bullous eruption, exfoliative dermatitis, hyperhidrosis, photosensitivity, pruritus, vasculitis, xerostomia

Busulfan

exanthem, urticaria, erythema multiforme minor, purpura, vasculitis, erythema nodosum, oral mucous membrane lesions, cheilitis, alopecia, induction of porphyria cutanea tarda, excessive dryness and fragility of skin, lupus erythematosus, macular erythema, anhidrosis, angioedema, *generalized (Addisonian) hyperpigmentation of skin* (on neck, upper trunk, nipples, abdomen, palmar creases and on mucous membranes)

Butorphanol

exanthem, *hyperhidrosis,* urticaria

Caffeine

pruritus, urticaria, hyperhidrosis

Calcitonin, human

flushing of face, ears, or hands, exanthem

Calcitonin, salmon

urticaria, local inflammation at injection site, flushing, pruritus of ear lobes

Calcium

flushing

Capreomycin sulfate

exanthem, urticaria

Captopril

exanthem, pruritus, flushing, purpura, pityriasis rosea-like eruption, lichenoid eruption, bullous pemphigoid, TEN, generalized hypersensitivity, pemphigus, atrophic glossitis, vasculitis, psoriasis, exfoliative dermatitis, oral mucosal lichenoid eruption, *angioedema,* photosensitivity, aphthous stomatitis, bullous eruption, ulcer on glans penis, hypermelanosis, *lupus erythematosus, diffuse alopecia, urticaria,* onycholysis

Carbamazepine

exanthem, pruritus, *urticaria,* angioedema, dermatitis, erythema multiforme minor, erythema multiforme major (Stevens-Johnson syndrome), vesicular or bullous eruption, TEN, purpura, vasculitis, erythema nodosum, lupus erythematosus, oral mucous membrane lesions, changes of skin color, fixed drug eruption, lichenoid eruption, facial and peripheral edema, alopecia, xerostomia, photosensitivity, photosensitivity with mycosis fungoides-like histology, generalized pustulation, exfoliative erythroderma, thrombocytopenic purpura, pseudolymphoma

Carbenicillin

exanthem, pruritus, *urticaria,* purpura

Carbidopa

exanthem, scleroderma-like cutaneous fibrosis, dermatomyositis-like exanthem

Carbinoxamine

fixed drug eruption, xerostomia, photosensitivity

Carboxymethylcellulose

angioedema

Carisoprodol

exanthem, pruritus, urticaria, angioedema, fixed drug eruption, erythema multiforme minor, purpura

Castor oil

angioedema, oral mucous membrane lesions, exanthem, urticaria

CCNU (Lomustine)

purpura, oral mucous membrane lesions, alopecia, exanthem

Cefaclor

exanthem, pruritus, *urticaria,* erythema multiforme minor, erythema multiforme major (Stevens-Johnson syndrome), TEN, oral ulceration, serum sickness-like syndrome

Cefadroxil

exanthem, pruritus, urticaria, angioedema, glossitis

Cefamandole

exanthem, pruritus, urticaria, angioedema, erythema multiforme minor, flushing with alcohol, vesicular or bullous eruption

Cefazolin

exanthem, pruritus, erythema multiforme major (Stevens-Johnson syndrome), urticaria, pustular eruption

Cefixime
exanthem, pruritus, urticaria, pustular eruption

Cefoperazone
exanthem, pruritus, *urticaria,* flushing with alcohol

Cefoxitin
exanthem, pruritus, exfoliative dermatitis, urticaria

Ceftazidime
exanthem, pruritus, angioedema, vesicular or bullous eruption, oral mucous membrane lesions, pustular eruption

Ceftriaxone
exanthem, pruritus, urticaria, anaphylaxis, serum sickness, hyperhidrosis, flushing, glossitis

Cefuroxime
exanthem, pruritus, urticaria, pustular exanthem, anaphylaxis

Cephalexin
exanthem, pruritus, urticaria, angioedema, oral mucous membrane lesions, dermatitis, erythema multiforme minor, erythema multiforme major (Stevens-Johnson syndrome), anaphylaxis, pustular exanthem

Chloral hydrate
exanthem, pruritus, urticaria, angioedema, fixed drug eruption, dermatitis, erythema multiforme minor, erythema multiforme major (Stevens-Johnson syndrome), vesicular or bullous eruption, purpura, vasculitis, oral mucous membrane lesions, lichenoid eruption, acneiform eruption, photosensitivity

Chlorambucil
exanthem, pruritus, urticaria, angioedema, exfoliative or eczematous dermatitis, TEN, oral mucous membrane lesions, alopecia, *herpes zoster,* erythema multiforme minor, pellagra-like eruption

Chloramphenicol
exanthem, pruritus, urticaria, angioedema, dermatitis, erythema multiforme minor, erythema multiforme major (Stevens-Johnson syndrome), vesicular or bullous eruption, TEN, purpura, vasculitis, lupus erythematosus, oral mucous membrane lesions, xerostomia, alopecia, pellagra-like reaction, photosensitivity, pustular eruption

Chlordiazepoxide
exanthem, pruritus, urticaria, angioedema, fixed drug eruption, dermatitis, erythema multiforme minor, purpura, vasculitis, erythema nodosum, lupus erythematosus, lichenoid eruption, alopecia, photosensitivity, exacerbation of porphyria cutanea tarda

Chlormezanone

exanthem, pruritus, fixed drug eruption, dermatitis, flushing, erythema multiforme minor, erythema multiforme major (Stevens-Johnson syndrome), TEN, xerostomia

Chloroquine

exanthem, lichenoid eruption, alopecia, acneiform eruption, depigmentation, angioedema, TEN, erythema multiforme minor, vasculitis, exfoliative dermatitis, hyperpigmentation, discoloration of hair and nails, oral mucous membrane lesions, *pruritus,* photosensitivity, lupus erythematosus, fixed drug eruption, urticaria, erythema annulare centrifugum, exacerbation of psoriasis, induction or exacerbation of porphyria cutanea tarda

Chlorotrianisene

urticaria, melasma, erythema multiforme minor, erythema nodosum, hemorrhagic eruption, alopecia, hirsutism

Chlorpheniramine

purpura, xerostomia, urticaria, exanthem

Chlorpromazine

dermatitis, miliaria-like eruption, *exanthem,* pruritus, urticaria, angioedema, fixed drug eruption, erythema multiforme minor, vesicular or bullous eruption, TEN, purpura, vasculitis, *lupus erythematosus (usually serologic changes only),* oral mucous membrane lesions, lichenoid eruption, hypertrichosis, exfoliative dermatitis, necrosis following injection, *photosensitivity,* contact dermatitis, photo-onycholysis, *brown or slate-gray or bluish to purple change in skin color in photoexposed areas*

Chlorpropamide

exanthem, pruritus, urticaria, dermatitis, erythema multiforme minor, erythema multiforme major (Stevens-Johnson syndrome), vesicular or bullous eruption, purpura, vasculitis, erythema nodosum, lupus erythematosus, oral mucous membrane lesions, alopecia, lichenoid eruption, photosensitivity, induction of porphyria cutanea tarda, exfoliative dermatitis, TEN, *flushing with ingestion of alcohol*

Chlorprothixene

exanthem, pruritus, angioedema, lupus erythematosus, oral mucous membrane lesions, dermatitis, urticarial reaction, photosensitivity

Chlortetracycline

exanthem, *pruritus,* urticaria, angioedema, fixed drug eruption, dermatitis, erythema multiforme minor, vesicular or bullous eruption, TEN, vasculitis, lupus erythematosus, *oral mucous membrane lesions,* onycholysis, *photosensitivity,* contact dermatitis, exfoliative dermatitis

Chlorthalidone

exanthem, urticaria, purpura, vasculitis, lupus erythematosus, TEN, photosensitivity, pseudoporphyria, psoriasiform eruption

Chlorzoxazone

exanthem, pruritus, urticaria, purpura, anaphylactoid reaction

Cholestyramine

exanthem, oral mucous membrane lesions, skin irritation, urticaria

Choline magnesium trisalicylate

erythema multiforme minor, urticaria, ecchymoses

Chorionic gonadotropin (HCG)

alopecia, edema, exanthem, urticaria, angioedema

Cimetidine

exanthem, urticaria, angioedema, erythema multiforme minor, acneiform eruption, TEN, exfoliative dermatitis, purpura, alopecia, pruritus, xerosis, relapse of lupus erythematosus, erythema, eczema, erythema annulare centrifugum, vasculitis, seborrheic-like dermatitis, induction of pustular, palmar psoriasis

Cinnarizine

lupus erythematosus, lichenoid eruption, vesicles

Ciprofloxacin

exanthem, pruritus, urticaria, photosensitivity, flushing, angioedema, cutaneous candidiasis, hyperpigmentation, erythema nodosum, erythema multiforme minor, TEN, vasculitis, purpura, vesicles, hyperhidrosis, erythroderma, anaphylactoid reaction, anaphylaxis, acneiform eruption

Cisplatin

angioedema, purpura, alopecia, *oral mucous membrane lesions,* "hypersensitivity reactions" that include "anxiety, flushing, burning, tingling, *pruritus,* cough, dyspnea, diaphoresis, *periorbital edema,* bronchospasm, vomiting, erythema, *urticaria, exanthem,* and hypotension"*

Clemastine

exanthem, pruritus, urticaria, photosensitivity

Clindamycin

exanthem - often morbilliform, *pruritus,* urticaria, angioedema, erythema multiforme minor, erythema multiforme major (Stevens-Johnson syndrome), xerosis, vasculitis, dermatitis, photosensitivity

---

* Weiss RB and Bruno S: Hypersensitivity reactions to cancer chemotherapeutic agents. *Annals Int Med.* 1981; 94:66-72.

Clofazimine

dermatitis, changes of skin and nail color (reddish blue, brown-red, slate gray), ichthyosis and xerosis, exanthem, pruritus, photosensitivity, erythroderma, acneiform eruption, monilial cheilitis, chromhidrosis

Clofibrate

exanthem, pruritus, urticaria, dermatitis, vesicular or bullous eruption, purpura, photosensitivity, lupus erythematosus, oral mucous membrane lesions, TEN, dry/brittle hair, alopecia, erythema multiforme minor, xerosis

Clomiphene

exanthem, urticaria, alopecia, *flushing,* allergic dermatitis, *hyperhidrosis*

Clonazepam

exanthem, angioedema, TEN, purpura, alopecia, hirsutism, ankle and facial edema

Clonidine

exanthem, pruritus, angioedema, vasculitis, oral mucous membrane lesions, mucosal pemphigoid, localized vesiculation, hyperpigmentation, excoriation, burning, pityriasis rosea-like eruption, xerostomia, Raynaud's phenomenon, psoriasis-like eruption, eczematous eruption, contact dermatitis, urticaria, alopecia

Clotrimazole

exanthem, urticaria

Codeine

exanthem, pruritus, urticaria, angioedema, fixed drug eruption, dermatitis, erythema multiforme minor, erythema multiforme major (Stevens-Johnson syndrome), vesicular or bullous eruption, TEN, purpura, vasculitis, erythema nodosum, photosensitivity, hyperhidrosis, exfoliative dermatitis

Colchicine

exanthem, pruritus, dermatitis, vesicular or bullous eruption, vasculitis, oral mucous membrane lesions, lichenoid eruption, *alopecia,* induction of porphyria cutanea tarda, urticaria, purpura

Colistin

exanthem, pruritus, urticaria

Compound Q

"rash," anaphylaxis

Copper

pruritus, urticaria, purpura, oral mucous membrane lesions, lichenoid eruption, photosensitivity

Cromolyn sodium

exanthem, pruritus, urticaria, angioedema, dermatitis, photosensitivity, lupus erythematosus, flushing, burning, erythema

Curare\Tubocurarine

exanthem, urticaria, angioedema

Cyclizine

urticaria, fixed drug eruption, exanthem

Cyclophosphamide

exanthem, urticaria, dermatitis, erythema multiforme minor, vesicular or bullous eruption, *TEN,* purpura, lichenoid eruption, acneiform eruption, *alopecia,* photosensitivity, *increased viral and fungal infections,* stomatitis, angioedema, anaphylaxis, vasculitis, benign and malignant skin tumors including dermatofibromas, miliaria-like eruption, palmar-plantar erythrodysesthesia syndrome, pruritus, *hyperpigmentation of skin, nails,* teeth and mucous membranes, nail ridging

Cycloserine

exanthem, pruritus, urticaria, dermatitis, oral mucous membrane lesions

Cyclosporine A

hypertrichosis, acneiform eruption, pruritus, pseudolymphoma, sebaceous hyperplasia, eruptive benign keratoses, aphthous stomatitis, exanthem, *cutaneous viral infections,* purpura, striae, urticaria, induction of various cutaneous malignancies, anaphylactoid reaction, *flushing,* psoriasiform eruption, coarseness of facial features in children, *gingival hyperplasia,* alopecia, hair breakage

Cyproheptadine

exanthem, angioedema, lichenoid eruption, urticaria, hyperhidrosis, xerostomia, photosensitivity

Cytarabine

exanthem, dermatitis, purpura, *oral mucous membrane lesions,* depigmentation, skin ulceration, freckling, *alopecia,* angioedema, pruritus, urticaria, palmar-plantar erythrodysesthesia, neutrophilic eccrine hidradenitis, syndrome of fever, malaise, arthralgias, conjunctivitis and maculopapular exanthem in 24 hours preventable with corticosteroids

Dacarbazine (DTIC®)

photosensitivity, exanthem, urticaria, angioedema, fixed drug eruption, hypermelanosis of nails, inflammation of actinic keratoses, *flushing,* anaphylaxis, localized infusion site reactions

Dactinomycin

exanthem, papular-pustular *acneiform eruption,* alopecia, erythema, *hyperpigmentation,* exfoliative dermatitis, dermatitis, erythema multiforme minor, TEN, *oral mucous membrane lesions,* pain, redness, swelling, chemical cellulitis on infusion, *radiation recall*

Danazol

exanthem, pruritus, acneiform eruption, hirsutism, edema, *alopecia, flushing,* hyperhidrosis, cholinergic urticaria, erythema multiforme minor, aggravation of lupus erythematosus, *seborrhea,* spider angiomas

Dantrolene

exanthem, acneiform eruption, abnormal hair growth, pruritus, urticaria, hyperhidrosis, eczematoid eruption, erythema

Dapsone

exanthem, pruritus, urticaria, *fixed drug eruption,* dermatitis, erythema multiforme minor, vesicular or bullous eruption, TEN, purpura, erythema nodosum, lupus erythematosus, lichenoid eruption, exfoliative dermatitis, erythroderma, isolated blisters or bullous eruption, photosensitivity, *hypermelanosis,* blue-gray change in *skin color* with methemaglobinemia (Dapsone hypersensitivity syndrome: exanthem, fever, adenopathy, hepatitis)

Daunorubicin

exanthem, urticaria, angioedema, *oral mucous membrane lesions, reversible alopecia,* brown to black nail bands, pain, redness, swelling at infusion site or distally, hypermelanosis

ddC (dideoxycytidine)

maculopapular eruption on day 10 or 11 of therapy, papulovesicular lesions, nail changes, *angioedema, erythroderma, vesicular or bullous eruption,* aphthous stomatitis, *lesions on soft palate, tongue and pharynx*

ddI (see didanosine)

Deferoxamine

exanthem, pruritus, urticaria, erythema, irritation, swelling and induration on injection

Demeclocycline

photosensitivity, exanthem, urticaria, angioedema, fixed drug eruption, dermatitis, vesicular or bullous eruption, lupus erythematosus, oral mucous membrane lesions, lichenoid eruption, acneiform eruption, onycholysis

Desipramine

exanthem, urticaria, *angioedema,* purpura, photodermatitis, petechiae, itching, alopecia, photosensitivity, hyperhidrosis, pruritus, flushing

Desmopressin

local erythema at injection site, facial flushing

Dexamethasone

urticaria, petechiae, *ecchymoses, acneiform eruption, hirsutism,* impaired wound healing, atrophic fragile skin, erythema, hyperhidrosis, allergic dermatitis, xerosis, folliculitis, hypertrichosis, hypopigmentation, *striae,* miliaria, necrosis following injection, pruritus

Dexbrompheniramine

exanthem

Dextran

exanthem, pruritus, urticaria, angioedema, dermatitis, purpura, fixed drug eruption, alopecia, flushing

Diazepam

exanthem, urticaria, angioedema, fixed drug eruption, dermatitis, vesicular or bullous eruption, purpura, vasculitis, acneiform eruption, photosensitivity, hypermelanosis of scars

Diazoxide

exanthem, *pruritus,* purpura, lichenoid eruption, hypermelanosis, alopecia, *hypertrichosis lanuginosa,* depigmentation, hirsutism, photosensitivity

Diclofenac

exanthem, pruritus, erythema nodosum, IgA-bullous dermatitis, aggravation of porphyria cutanea tarda, TEN, alopecia, urticaria, dermatitis, erythema multiforme major (Stevens-Johnson syndrome), angioedema, exfoliative dermatitis, pustular psoriasis, aphthous stomatitis, hyperhidrosis, photosensitivity, purpura

Dicumarol

skin necrosis, alopecia, urticaria, dermatitis, "purple toes"

Didanosine (ddI)

exanthem, pruritus, hyperhidrosis, xerostomia, eczematous eruption, flushing, erythema multiforme major (Stevens-Johnson syndrome); in children as in adults plus impetigo, excoriation, erythema

Diethylstilbestrol

exanthem, pruritus, angioedema, fixed drug eruption, vesicular or bullous eruption, purpura, vasculitis, melasma, erythema multiforme minor, erythema nodosum, alopecia, hirsutism, hypertrichosis, acanthosis nigricans, photosensitivity, exacerbation of porphyria cutanea tarda

Diflunisal

exanthem, erythema multiforme minor, erythema multiforme major (Stevens-Johnson syndrome), exfoliative dermatitis, urticaria, pruritus, stomatitis, photosensitivity, vasculitis, onycholysis, hyperhidrosis, TEN, erythroderma, xerostomia

Digoxin

fixed drug eruption, isolated blisters or bullous eruption, purpura, vasculitis, exanthem, exacerbation of psoriasis, erythema multiforme major (Stevens-Johnson syndrome)

Diltiazem

erythema multiforme minor, erythema multiforme major (Stevens-Johnson syndrome), gingival hyperplasia, TEN, erythromelalgia, lupus erythematosus-like exanthem, psoriasiform exanthem, purpura, vasculitis, exfoliative dermatitis in a patient with psoriasis, *exanthem,* pruritus, flushing, pustular eruption

Dimenhydrinate

fixed drug eruption, vasculitis

Dimercaprol

urticaria, vesicular or bullous eruption, oral mucous membrane lesions, burning sensation

Diphenhydramine

exanthem, pruritus, urticaria, fixed drug eruption, dermatitis, vasculitis, hyperhidrosis, TEN, xerostomia, photosensitivity, contact dermatitis

Diphenidol

exanthem, xerostomia

Diphenoxylate

exanthem, pruritus, urticaria, angioedema, *oral mucous membrane lesions* and swelling of gums

Dipyridamole

exanthem, erythema multiforme minor, flushing, pruritus

Disopyramide

exanthem, pruritus, photosensitivity, purpura, alopecia, angioedema, vasculitis, xerostomia

Disulfiram

exanthem, pruritus, urticaria, fixed drug eruption, dermatitis, vesicular or bullous eruption, purpura, vasculitis, acneiform eruption, lupus erythematosus, flushing with ethanol ingestion, exacerbation of porphyria cutanea tarda, pustular dermatitis, polyarteritis nodosa-like syndrome

Dopamine

piloerection, Raynaud's phenomenon

Doxapram

pruritus, flushing, hyperhidrosis

Doxepin

exanthem, pruritus, purpura, hyperhidrosis, edema, photosensitization, flushing, alopecia, xerostomia

Doxorubicin

exanthem, urticaria, dermatitis, vesicular or bullous eruption, purpura, *reversible alopecia,* necrosis after injection, onycholysis, flushing, erythema, *stomatitis,* hyperpigmentation of skin, *hypermelanosis of nails,* radiation recall, chemical cellulitis and phlebitis, *urticarial flare proximal to injection site,* inflammation of actinic keratoses, palmar-plantar erythrodysesthesia syndrome

Doxycycline

exanthem, urticaria, fixed drug eruption, dermatitis, oral mucous membrane lesions, onycholysis, *photosensitivity,* angioedema, exfoliative dermatitis, aggravation of lupus erythematosus

DTIC - see Dacarbazine

Edrophonium

hyperhidrosis

EDTA (edathamil)

angioedema, dermatitis, oral mucous membrane lesions

Enalapril (lower rate of reactions than with Captopril)

exanthem, pruritus, urticaria, angioedema, TEN, exfoliative dermatitis, erythema multiforme minor, erythema multiforme major (Stevens-Johnson syndrome), vasculitis, photosensitivity, *lupus erythematosus,* oral mucous membrane lesions, anaphylaxis, flushing, hyperhidrosis, alopecia, pemphigus folaceus, induction or aggravation of psoriasis

Enflurane

anaphylactoid reaction

Enoxacin

exanthem, *urticaria,* photosensitivity, dermatitis, hyperhidrosis, TEN, erythema multiforme major (Stevens-Johnson syndrome)

Ephedrine

exanthem, urticaria, fixed drug eruption, dermatitis, vesicular or bullous eruption, purpura, vasculitis, hyperhidrosis, dry nose and throat

Epinephrine

urticaria, fixed drug eruption, hyperhidrosis, pallor, wheal and hemorrhage at injection site, xerostomia

Erythrityl tetranitrate

exanthem, vasculitis, exfoliative dermatitis

Erythromycin

exanthem, pruritus, urticaria, angioedema, fixed drug eruption, purpura, oral mucous membrane lesions, xerosis, desquamation, erythema, burning sensation, TEN, acneiform eruption

Erythropoietin

exanthem, pruritus, urticaria, *angioedema,* exacerbation of acne

Estradiol

in transdermal delivery system: erythema, pruritus, *dermatitis,* pustules, hypermelanosis after UVB at the site of application

Estramustine phosphate

exanthem, pruritus, easy bruising, flushing, thinning hair, xerosis

Estrogens

urticaria, lupus erythematosus, *melasma,* alopecia, hypertrichosis, hirsutism, erythema multiforme minor, erythema nodosum, hemorrhagic eruption, induction of porphyria cutanea tarda, fixed drug eruption, acneiform eruption, striae distensae, pruritus, gingival hyperplasia, patchy livedo, acanthosis nigricans-like eruption

Ethacrynic acid

exanthem, purpura, vasculitis, lupus erythematosus

Ethambutol

exanthem, pruritus, alopecia, urticaria, dermatitis, purpura, lupus erythematosus, hyperhidrosis, exfoliative dermatitis, lichenoid eruption, TEN

Ethchlorvynol

exanthem, urticaria, fixed drug eruption, purpura

Ethinyl estradiol + Ethynodiol diacetate

erythema nodosum, lupus erythematosus, edema, exanthem, alopecia

Ethinyl estradiol + Megestrol acetate

erythema multiforme minor, lupus erythematosus, erythema nodosum, alopecia

Ethinyl estradiol + Norgestrel

dermatitis, edema, exanthem, lupus erythematosus, erythema nodosum, erythema multiforme minor

Ethionamide

exanthem, *urticaria,* dermatitis, purpura, lupus erythematosus, oral mucous membrane lesions, alopecia, xerostomia, photosensitivity, pellagra-like reaction with lilac-brown color, *acne,* ichthyosiform eruption

Ethosuximide

exanthem, pruritus, urticaria, angioedema, erythema multiforme minor, erythema multiforme major (Stevens-Johnson syndrome), purpura, lupus erythematosus, hirsutism

Ethotoin

exanthem, pruritus, urticaria, angioedema, fixed drug eruption, dermatitis, vesicular or bullous eruption, purpura, oral mucous membrane lesions

Etidronate

exanthem, pruritus, urticaria, angioedema

Etodolac

exanthem, angioedema, hyperhidrosis, urticaria, vasculitis, erythema multiforme major (Stevens-Johnson syndrome), vesiculobullous eruption, exfoliative dermatitis

Etoposide - VP16

exanthem, pruritus, *oral mucous membrane lesions,* reversible *alopecia,* scaling, anaphylaxis, xerosis, radiation recall, erythema multiforme major (Stevens-Johnson syndrome), acne

Etretinate

alopecia, palmar-plantar desquamation, *xerosis of skin/nasal mucosa and conjunctivae,* stomatitis, epistaxis, *eczematous dermatitis,* itching, red scaly face, *skin fragility,* bruising, *cheilitis, pruritus,* hair thinning, photosensitivity, erythema multiforme-like eruption, edema, exuberant granulation tissue, bullous eruption, herpes simplex, *nail dystrophy,* paronychia, hyperhidrosis

Famotidine

alopecia, acne, pruritus, xerosis, flushing, contact eczema, vasculitis, exanthem, urticaria, angioedema, anaphylaxis, pustular eruption

Fansidar

erythema multiforme major (Stevens-Johnson syndrome), erythroderma, exanthem, photosensitivity, TEN, oral lichenoid eruption

Felodipine

exanthem, *flushing,* hyperhidrosis

Fenbufen

exanthem, pruritus, urticaria, facial edema, TEN, erythema multiforme minor, purpura, vasculitis, erythroderma, lichenoid eruption

Fenfluramine

exanthem, pruritus, urticaria, alopecia, xerostomia

Fenoprofen

exanthem, pruritus, urticaria, purpura, acneiform eruption, erythema multiforme minor, TEN, exfoliative dermatitis, angioedema, vesiculobullous eruption, xerostomia, hyperhidrosis

Fibrinolysin

urticaria, angioedema, itching, burning

Filgrastim (G-CSF)

Sweet's syndrome-like reaction

Fluconazole

exanthem, erythema multiforme major (Stevens-Johnson syndrome {patients taking other medications, however}), anaphylaxis, pruritus, purpura

Flucytosine

exanthem, urticaria, purpura

Fluorescein

pruritus, urticaria, purpura, photosensitivity

5-Fluorouracil

exanthem, pruritus, angioedema, dermatitis, vesicular or bullous eruption, lichenoid eruption, *alopecia,* telangiectasia, scarring, xerosis, fissuring, palmar-plantar erythrodysethesia, *photosensitivity,* TEN, bullous pemphigoid, serpentine (postinflammatory) hyperpigmentation along injected veins, isolated blisters or bullous eruption, *hypermelanosis in photodistribution,* pigmented macules, stomatitis, hyperpigmentation of nails, inflammation of actinic keratoses

Fluoxetine

exanthem, pruritus, urticaria, angioedema, dermatitis, erythema multiforme minor, purpura, lupus erythematosus, *hyperhidrosis, xerostomia, flushing,* serum sickness, acne, alopecia, psoriasiform eruption, xerosis, subcutaneous nodules, aphthous stomatitis, gingivitis, glossitis

Fluoxymesterone

exanthem, purpura, acneiform eruption, hirsutism, androgenetic alopecia, seborrhea, acne

Fluphenazine

exanthem, pruritus, urticaria, angioedema, dermatitis, purpura, vasculitis, photodermatitis, seborrhea, exfoliative dermatitis, *hyperhidrosis,* acrocyanosis

Flurazepam

exanthem, pruritus

Flurbiprofen

exanthem, pruritus, angioedema, urticaria, eczema, photosensitivity, TEN, exfoliative dermatitis, xerosis, alopecia, hyperhidrosis, oral lichenoid eruption, vasculitis

Folic acid

exanthem, pruritus, urticaria, dermatitis, acneiform eruption

Foscarnet

Genital and oral ulcerations, fixed drug eruption, phlebitis at infusion site

Furosemide

exanthem, pruritus, urticaria, dermatitis, erythema multiforme minor, vesicular or bullous eruption, purpura, vasculitis, lichenoid eruption, exfoliative dermatitis, bullous pemphigoid, pustular eruption, pseudoporphyria, photosensitivity, Sweet's syndrome-like eruption, epidermolysis bullosa *acquisita-like* eruption, pustular eruption

Ganciclovir

exanthem, alopecia

G-CSF - see Filgrastim

Gemfibrozil

exanthem, eczema, pruritus, urticaria, exacerbation of psoriasis, hyperhidrosis, vasculitis, exfoliative dermatitis

Gentamicin

exanthem, pruritus, urticaria, purpura, alopecia, erythema, dermatitis, photosensitivity, necrosis at injection site

Glipizide

exanthem, erythema, urticaria, pruritus, eczema, flushing

Globulin, immune: Human

local pain/tenderness at injection site, urticaria, angioedema, flushing

Glucagon

urticaria, angioedema, dermatitis, erythema multiforme minor, flushing, necrolytic migratory erythema

Glutethimide

exanthem, pruritus, urticaria, fixed drug eruption, erythema multiforme minor, erythema multiforme major (Stevens-Johnson syndrome), vesicular or bullous eruption, purpura, vasculitis, lupus erythematosus, blotchy hyperpigmentation, xerostomia

Glyburide

exanthem, pruritis, urticaria, angioedema, vasculitis, erythema

GM-CSF (granulocyte macrophage colony stimulating factor)

lupus erythematosus, red pruritic skin at injection site, *generalized pruritus,* *exanthem,* flushing, angioedema, erythema, erythroderma, papules, epidermolysis bullosa acquisita, pemphigus, alopecia, Sweet's syndrome-like eruption

Gold

exanthem, pruritus, urticaria, fixed drug eruption, *eczematous dermatitis,* erythema multiforme minor, *vesicular or bullous eruption,* TEN, purpura, vasculitis, erythema nodosum, photodermatitis, lupus erythematosus, *oral mucous membrane lesions,* lichenoid eruption, blue-gray or yellowish changes in skin color, chrysiasis, discoloration of nails, alopecia, acneiform eruption, exfoliative dermatitis, stomatitis, erythroderma, pyoderma gangrenosum, photosensitivity, nonspecific papules and plaques, pityriasis rosea-like eruption, porphyria cutanea tarda, granuloma annulare, seborrheic dermatitis, pemphigus, psoriasiform eruption, angiofibromas on trunk, erythema annulare centrifugum

Griseofulvin

exanthem, pruritus, urticaria, angioedema, fixed drug eruption, dermatitis, erythema multiforme minor, erythema multiforme major (Stevens-Johnson syndrome), vesicular or bullous eruption, purpura, vasculitis, photodermatitis, lupus erythematosus, oral mucous membrane lesions, lichenoid eruption, changes of skin color, alopecia, pityriasis rosea-like eruption, porphyria cutanea tarda, exacerbation of lupus erythematosus, photosensitivity, TEN, exfoliative dermatitis, flushing

Guanethidine

exanthem, fixed drug eruption, vasculitis, lupus erythematosus, alopecia, dermatitis, polyarteritis nodosa-like syndrome

Haloperidol

exanthem, urticaria, alopecia, acneiform eruption, depigmentation, photosensitivity, seborrheic dermatitis

Halothane

exanthem, urticaria, angioedema, alopecia

Heparin

exanthem, pruritus, urticaria, angioedema, purpura, *alopecia,* erythema, itching, burning, necrosis, onycholysis, allergic erythematous plaques, eczema-like erythematous plaques, vasculitis; at injection site: hematoma, infection, necrosis, red plaques and patches

Hyaluronidase

urticaria, angioedema, exanthem, anaphylaxis

Hydralazine

exanthem, urticaria, angioedema, dermatitis, purpura, vasculitis, photosensitivity, *lupus erythematosus,* oral and genital mucous membrane ulcers, flushing, pruritus, fixed drug eruption, erythema multiforme minor, erythema multiforme major (Stevens-Johnson syndrome), pyoderma gangrenosum-like ulcers, Sweet's syndrome, erythema nodosum

Hydrochlorothiazide

exanthem, pruritus, urticaria, dermatitis, erythema multiforme minor, erythema multiforme major (Stevens-Johnson syndrome), vesicular or bullous eruption, TEN, purpura, vasculitis, lichenoid eruption, changes of skin color, photosensitivity, lupus erythematosus, ichthyosiform eruption, erythema annulare centrifugum-like eruption

Hydrocortisone

pruritus, urticaria, angioedema, purpura, vasculitis, impaired wound healing, fragile skin, petechiae, ecchymoses, facial erythema, hyperhidrosis, folliculitis, hypertrichosis, *acneiform eruption,* hypopigmentation, *striae, hirsutism, acneiform eruption*

Hydroxychloroquine

exanthem, pruritus, urticaria, purpura, vasculitis, photodermatitis, bleaching of hair color, alopecia, skin and mucosal pigmentation, TEN, exacerbation of psoriasis, exfoliative dermatitis, erythema annulare centrifugum

Hydroxyurea

exanthem, pruritus, fixed drug eruption, dermatitis, erythema multiforme minor, vasculitis, oral mucous membrane lesions, lichenoid eruption, hypermelanosis, facial edema, brown discoloration of nails and rare pigmented longitudinal nail bands, dermatomyositis-like syndrome, alopecia, skin and subcutaneous atrophy, skin ulcerations, skin cancers in photoexposed areas

Hydroxyzine

exanthem, pruritus, urticaria, angioedema, dermatitis, erythema multiforme minor, xerostomia

Ibuprofen

exanthem, pruritus, urticaria, angioedema, erythema multiforme minor, erythema multiforme major (Stevens-Johnson syndrome), purpura, vasculitis, lupus erythematosus, oral mucous membrane lesions, alopecia, TEN, photosensitivity, fixed drug eruption, exacerbation of psoriasis, exfoliative dermatitis, bullous pemphigoid-like eruption, bullae on legs, anaphylactoid reaction

Imipenem-cilastin

exanthem, pruritus, urticaria, angioedema, erythema multiforme minor, TEN, pustular eruption

Imipramine

urticaria, *exanthem, pruritus,* angioedema, fixed drug eruption, dermatitis, purpura, lupus erythematosus, oral mucous membrane lesions, lichenoid eruption, petechiae, alopecia, peripheral edema, *xerostomia, hyperhidrosis,* photosensitivity, hyperpigmentation, exfoliative dermatitis, flushing

Indapamide

exanthem, pruritus, urticaria, vasculitis

Indomethacin

exanthem, pruritus, urticaria, angioedema, vesicular or bullous eruption, TEN, purpura, vasculitis, erythema nodosum, *oral mucous membrane lesions,* changes of skin color, alopecia, pemphigus, lichenoid eruption, flushing, aggravation of psoriasis, periorbital edema, photosensitivity, erythema multiforme minor, eczematous eruption, exacerbation of dermatitis herpetiformis, hyperhidrosis

Insulin

exanthem, pruritus, urticaria, angioedema, vesicular or bullous eruption, purpura, vasculitis, lupus erythematosus; at injection site: redness, swelling, pruritus, lipoatrophy or lipohypertrophy, fascial cicatrix, mesenchymoma

Interferon alpha (2a or 2b)

exanthem, pruritus, alopecia, purpura, hypertrichosis, increased growth of eyelashes, systemic sclerosis, bleeding gums or *sore gums, xerostomia,* edema, *xerosis,* cyanosis, flushing of the skin, Raynaud's phenomenon, urticaria, exacerbation or induction of psoriasis or herpes, acne, fungal infection, eczematous eruption, telangiectasia, photosensitivity, erythema\transient urticaria at injection site

Interferon gamma

exanthem, hyperhidrosis

Interleukin 2 (Aldesleukin)

local reaction at injection site, erythroderma with necrotic lesions and purpura or tense blisters, mucositis, glossitis, punctate superficial ulcers, erosions in scars, erythrodermic flares of psoriasis, icterus, erythema nodosum, basal cell carcinoma and other tumors at injection site, alopecia, macular erythema with burning and pruritus on head, neck and chest, pemphigus, erythema, *exanthem,* petechiae on legs, facial/palmar-plantar edema, urticarial papules, urticaria, cutaneous toxicity in 96% of patients and 72% of cycles within 36-72h—recurrences may be earlier but milder on subsequent cycles

Iodine

acneiform eruption, iododerma, angioedema, erythema multiforme minor, erythema nodosum, exfoliative dermatitis, dermatitis, contact dermatitis, alopecia, fixed drug eruption, isolated blisters or bullous eruption, lichenoid eruption

Ipodate

exanthem, pruritus, urticaria, purpura

Iron - Ferrous gluconate sulfate

changes of skin color (hemochromatosis), exacerbation of porphyria cutanea tarda, exanthem, urticaria, vasculitis; at injection site: brown discoloration

Isocarboxazid

exanthem, pruritus, angioedema, vasculitis, oral mucous membrane lesions, peripheral edema, photosensitivity

Isoniazid (INH)

exanthem, *pruritus, urticaria,* angioedema, dermatitis, erythema multiforme minor, vesicular or bullous eruption, TEN, purpura, vasculitis, *lupus erythematosus, oral mucous membrane lesions,* alopecia, hypertrichosis, acneiform eruption, exfoliative dermatitis, lichenoid eruption, purpura, acne, onycholysis, pellagra-like eruption, photosensitivity, pustular eruption

Isoproterenol

flushing/hyperhidrosis, oral mucous membrane lesions

Isosorbide dinitrate

exanthem, dermatitis, cutaneous vasodilation with flushing, exfoliative dermatitis

Isotretinoin

xerosis, *skin fragility, pruritus, dry nasal or oral mucosa, conjunctivitis, cheilitis, epistaxis, peeling of fingertips/desquamation* generally, thinning hair, erythema multiforme minor, erythema nodosum, flushing, exuberant granulation tissue, pityriasis rosea-like eruption, vasculitis, eruptive xanthoma, leukoderma, hyperpigmentation, *eczematous dermatitis, photosensitivity,* urticaria, *alopecia,* hypertrichosis, *purpura,* pyogenic granuloma-like lesions, scalp folliculitis, pyoderma gangrenosum

Isradipine

exanthem, edema, *flushing, pruritus,* urticaria, *xerostomia*

Itraconazole

exanthem, pruritus, xerostomia, conjuctivitis, edema

Kanamycin

exanthem, pruritus, lupus erythematosus, oral mucous membrane lesions, dermatitis

Ketamine

exanthem, transient erythema and morbilliform exanthem, porphyria variegata

Ketoconazole

urticaria, anaphylaxis, *dermatitis,* exfoliative dermatitis, irritation, alopecia, abnormal hair texture, scalp pustules, xerosis, *pruritus,* fixed drug eruption, photodermatitis, *exanthem,* hyperpigmentation

Ketoprofen

exanthem, pruritus, urticaria, angioedema, dermatitis, oral mucous membrane lesions, alopecia, purpura, hyperhidrosis, bullous exanthem, exfoliative dermatitis, photosensitivity, discoloration, onycholysis, xerostomia, anaphylactoid reaction, anaphylaxis, palmar erythema

Ketorolac

pruritus, urticaria

Labetalol

pruritus, dermatitis, vesicular or bullous eruption, purpura, lichenoid eruption, Raynaud's phenomenon, *flushing,* pityriasis rosea-like eruption, angioedema, exanthem, lupus erythematosus, induction of psoriasis, urticaria, alopecia, anaphylaxis

L-Dopa - see Levodopa

Levamisole

exanthem, pruritus, *urticaria,* angioedema, vesicular or bullous eruption, vasculitis, *oral mucous membrane lesions,* lichenoid eruption, dermatitis, alopecia, lupus erythematosus, *erythema multiforme minor, erythema nodosum*

Levodopa

exanthem, urticaria, purpura, changes of skin color, alopecia, *flushing,* hyperhidrosis, aggravation of lupus erythematosus, pemphigus

Levonorgestrel

hirsutism, alopecia, erythema multiforme minor, erythema nodosum, acne, edema, blisters, exacerbation of psoriasis

Levothyroxine

alopecia, exacerbation of acne vulgaris

Lidocaine (reactions are rare and often due to preservatives)

urticaria, edema, bullae, exanthem, pruritus, angioedema, dermatitis, papulovesicular eruption. No reactions reported to intravenous lidocaine.

Lincomycin

exanthem, pruritus, urticaria, angioedema, vesicular or bullous eruption, purpura, oral mucous membrane lesions, photosensitivity, exfoliative dermatitis

Lisinopril

exanthem, pruritus, angioedema, vasculitis, flushing

Lithium

exanthem, *pruritus,* vesicular or bullous eruption, vasculitis, oral mucous membrane lesions, *alopecia,* acneiform eruption, acne, chronic folliculitis, *psoriasis or psoriasiform eruption,* cutaneous ulcers, angioedema, exfoliative dermatitis, pretibial and ankle edema, *lupus erythematosus* (usually positive ANA), exacerbation of Darier's disease, angular cheilitis, *eczematous dermatitis,* keratoderma, prurigo nodularis, pustular eruption, seborrheic dermatitis—worsened or improved, urticaria, onychodystrophy, xerosis, *ichthyosiform eruption,* erythema multiforme minor

Loperamide

exanthem, erythema nodosum, xerostomia, gingivitis

Loratadine

urticaria, angioedema

Lorazepam

exanthem

Lovastatin

exanthem, pruritus, alopecia and a rare hypersensitivity syndrome accompanied by various featrures including anaphylaxis, angioedema, lupus-like syndrome (with positive ANA), vasculitis, purpura, urticaria, photosensitivity, flushing, TEN, erythema multiforme major (Stevens-Johnson syndrome)

Loxapine

xerostomia, hyperhidrosis, dermatitis, exanthem, flushing, seborrhea, alopecia, pruritus

Lypressin

periorbital edema, itching

Magnesium

fixed drug eruption, dermatitis, oral mucous membrane lesions

Mannitol

urticaria

Maprotiline

exanthem, urticaria, xerostomia, hyperhidrosis, acneiform eruption, erythema multiforme minor, flushing, pruritus, purpura, vasculitis

Mechlorethamine (Mustine)

erythema multiforme minor, squamous cell carcinoma, bullae, purpura, alopecia, exanthem, telangiectasia, *contact dermatitis,* hyperpigmentation with topical use, immediate hypersensitivity reaction.

Meclofenamate

exanthem, fixed drug eruption, aggravated psoriasis, urticaria, *pruritus,* erythema multiforme minor, erythema multiforme major (Stevens-Johnson syndrome), exfoliative dermatitis, vasculitis, purpura, petechiae, vesiculobullous eruption, photosensitivity, erythema nodosum

Mefenamic acid

exanthem, urticaria, angioedema, pruritus, fixed drug eruption, facial edema, bullous pemphigoid, purpura, vasculitis, anaphylactoid reaction

Melphalan

exanthem, vasculitis, oral mucous membrane lesions, alopecia, angioedema, anaphylaxis, hypermelanosis of nails, urticaria, pruritus

Menthol

urticaria, angioedema, fixed drug eruption, dermatitis, vasculitis, exanthem

Meperidine

exanthem, pruritus, urticaria, angioedema, purpura, TEN, photosensitivity; at injection site: panniculitis, scleroderma-like lesions, wheal and flare over vein with IV administration

Mephenytoin

exanthem, pruritus, urticaria, angioedema, dermatitis, erythema multiforme minor, vesicular or bullous eruption, TEN, purpura, vasculitis, lupus erythematosus, melasma-like or Addisonian changes in skin color, exfoliative dermatitis, alopecia, gingival hyperplasia, polyarteritis nodosa-like syndrome

Mepivacaine

urticaria, angioedema, vesicular or bullous eruption, pruritus, hyperhidrosis

Meprobamate

exanthem, pruritus, *urticaria,* angioedema, fixed drug eruption, dermatitis, erythema multiforme minor, erythema multiforme major (Stevens-Johnson syndrome), vesicular or bullous eruption, TEN, purpura, vasculitis, erythema nodosum, lupus erythematosus, peripheral edema, xerostomia, photosensitivity, exacerbation of porphyria cutanea tarda, Addisonian hypermelanosis, stomatitis, pityriasis rosea-like eruption, exfoliative dermatitis, anaphylaxis

Mercaptopurine

exanthem, dermatitis, TEN, lupus erythematosus, *oral mucous membrane lesions,* hyperpigmentation, photosensitivity, pellagra-like eruption, lichenoid eruption, alopecia

Mercury

exanthem, pruritus, urticaria, angioedema, fixed drug eruption, dermatitis, erythema multiforme minor, vesicular or bullous eruption, purpura, oral mucous membrane lesions, lichenoid eruption, alopecia, acneiform eruption, depigmentation, photosensitivity, lupus erythematosus, exfoliative dermatitis, contact dermatitis, pink disease (acrodynia), blue-black perifollicular pigmentation

Mesna

exanthem, urticaria, angioedema, fixed drug eruption, erythroderma, bullae, mucosal lesions

Mesoridazine

exanthem, pruritus, angioedema, hypertrophic papillae of tongue, photosensitivity

Mestranol

photosensitivity, edema, exanthem, *melasma,* lupus erythematosus, erythema nodosum

Mestranol + Norethindrone

urticaria, erythema nodosum, photosensitivity, erythema multiforme minor, melasma, gingival hyperplasia, herpes gestationis

Methadone

exanthem, pruritus, urticaria, angioedema, *hyperhidrosis*

Methamphetamine

exanthem, urticaria, fixed drug eruption, alopecia, acneiform eruption, xerostomia, lupus erythematosus; at injection site: granulomas, hyperpigmentation, scar, slough

Methantheline bromide

exanthem, dermatitis, xerosis

Methaqualone

fixed drug eruption, erythema multiforme major (Stevens-Johnson syndrome), exanthem, pruritus, urticaria, brown discoloration of tongue

Methenamine

exanthem, urticaria, angioedema, fixed drug eruption, dermatitis, erythema multiforme minor, lichenoid eruption

Methenamine-hippurate

exanthem, fixed drug eruption

Methenamine-mandelate

exanthem

Methicillin
exanthem, pruritus, *urticaria,* vesicular or bullous eruption, oral mucous membrane lesions

Methimazole
exanthem, pruritus, *urticaria,* purpura, lupus erythematosus, alopecia, edema, hypermelanosis

Methohexital
exanthem, urticaria, angioedema, pruritus, erythema

Methotrexate
exanthem, pruritus, urticaria, eczematous dermatitis, TEN, purpura, vasculitis, *photosensitivity,* acneiform eruption, depigmentation, hyperpigmentation, ecchymoses, telangiectasia, acne, *various cutaneous infections,* discoloration of nails, induction of porphyria cutanea tarda, erythema multiforme minor, stomatitis, *alopecia,* angioedema, exfoliative erythroderma, squamous cell carcinoma, epidermal necrosis and cutaneous ulcers, vesiculation and ulceration over pressure areas, anaphylactoid reaction, Raynaud's phenomenon, paronychia, reactivation of radiation dermatitis and sunburn, palmar-plantar erythrodysesthesia

Methoxsalen + ultraviolet A (UVA) light (PUVA)
exanthem, pruritus, dermatitis, vesicular or bullous eruption, *lupus erythematosus* (positive ANA), *hypertrichosis,* acneiform eruption, hypopigmentation, edema, miliaria, urticaria, *photosensitivity,* isolated blisters or bullous eruption, alopecia, *lentigines,* cutaneous neoplasms

Methyldopa
exanthem, pruritus, fixed drug eruption, dermatitis, erythema multiforme minor, purpura, *lupus erythematosus* (mostly serologic changes), oral mucous membrane lesions, hypermelanosis, TEN, lichenoid eruption, xerostomia, photosensitivity, seborrheic dermatitis, urticaria, alopecia, vasculitis

Methylphenidate
exanthem, urticaria, erythema multiforme minor, purpura, vasculitis, photosensitivity, alopecia

Methylprednisolone
urticaria, angioedema, *acneiform eruption,* impaired wound healing, fragile skin, petechiae, *ecchymoses,* facial erythema, hyperhidrosis, alopecia, *hirsutism, striae*

Methysergide (maleate)
exanthem, dermatitis, lupus erythematosus, changes of skin color: hypermelanosis/thickened reddish "orange-peel skin," alopecia, facial flush, telangiectasia, peripheral edema, Raynaud's phenomenon

Metoclopramide
exanthem, urticaria, angioedema

Metolazone

exanthem, pruritus, vasculitis, xerosis

Metoprolol tartrate

exanthem, pruritus, induction or worsening of psoriasis, lupus erythematosus, psoriasiform eruption, exanthem, alopecia, dermatitis

Metronidazole

exanthem, pruritus, urticaria, fixed drug eruption, oral mucous membrane lesions: glossitis, stomatitis, xerostomia. Flushing after ingestion of ethanol, dryness of vagina or vulva, pityriasis rosea-like eruption, thrombophlebitis at injection site

Mexiletine

exanthem, nonspecific *edema,* alopecia

Miconazole

exanthem, pruritus, purpura, urticaria, thrombophlebitis at injection site

Minocycline

exanthem, pruritus, urticaria, fixed drug eruption, dermatitis, oral mucous membrane lesions, *pigmentation of skin (often pretibial) and mucous membranes,* postacne osteoma cutis, erythema nodosum, discoloration of teeth in adults as well as children, angioedema, erythema multiforme major (Stevens-Johnson syndrome), exfoliative dermatitis, lupus erythematosus, photosensitivity reported but not likely, Sweet's syndrome, onycholysis, anaphylaxis

Minoxidil

exanthem, *hypertrichosis,* hirsutism, pruritus, ankle edema, isolated blisters or bullous eruption, erythema multiforme major (Stevens-Johnson syndrome), lupus erythematosus

Misoprostol

exanthem

Mithramycin

exanthem, TEN, *purpura, oral mucous membrane lesions;* facial erythema and edema followed by desquamation and hyperpigmentation (an early indication of systemic toxicity)

Mitomycin C

exanthem, pruritus, angioedema, dermatitis, purpura, stomatitis, *alopecia,* necrosis/sloughing if drug is extravasated during injection, erythema, contact allergic dermatitis, urticaria, vesicular eruption with pruritus

Morphine

exanthem, *pruritus,* urticaria, angioedema, *xerostomia,* dermatitis, vesicular or bullous eruption, edema, diaphoresis, hyperhidrosis, wheals and/or local tissue irritation including bullae, panniculitis at injection site

Nafcillin
exanthem, pruritus, *urticaria*

Nalidixic acid
exanthem, changes of skin color (hyper- and hypomelanosis), alopecia, pruritus, urticaria, angioedema, photosensitivity, pseudoporphyria, erythema multiforme minor, lupus erythematosus, TEN, isolated blisters or bullous eruption, purpura, anaphylactoid reaction

Naproxen
exanthem, pruritus, urticaria, angioedema, purpura, oral mucous membrane lesions, pseudoporphyria, photosensitivity, vasculitis, vesiculobullous eruption, alopecia, fixed drug eruption, erythema multiforme minor, lichenoid eruption, hyperhidrosis, pustular eruption, anaphylactoid reaction, acneiform eruption

Neomycin
exanthem, pruritus, angioedema, dermatitis, vesicular or bullous eruption, TEN, oral mucous membrane lesions, isolated blisters or bullous eruption

Niacin - see Vitamin B3

Nicardipine
exanthem, flushing, edema, erythromelalgia

Nickel
exanthem, urticaria, dermatitis, vesicular or bullous eruption, contact dermatitis

Nicotinamide (niacinamide)
flushing and other cutaneous effects less common than with nicotinic acid

Nicotinic acid (Niacin)
flushing, dryness, pruritus, hypermelanosis and *acanthosis nigricans-like eruption,* xerosis, fixed drug eruption, pellagra-like eruption, exanthem, alopecia, urticaria

Nifedipine
exanthem, dermatitis, *flushing,* periorbital angioedema, erythema multiforme minor, erythema multiforme major (Stevens-Johnson syndrome), exfoliative erythroderma, psoriasiform exanthem, purpura, pruritus, urticaria, hyperhidrosis, edema, *gingival hyperplasia,* erythromelalgia, photosensitivity, fixed drug/bullous fixed drug eruption, alopecia, erythema nodosum

Nimodipine
exanthem, edema

Nitrofurantoin

alopecia, exfoliative dermatitis, erythema multiforme minor, angioedema, bullae, TEN, erythema nodosum, lupus erythematosus, purpura, pruritus, flushing, urticaria, fixed drug eruption, isolated blisters or bullous eruption, exanthem, eczematous eruption, photosensitivity, anaphylaxis

Nitroglycerin

exanthem, urticaria, dermatitis, purpura, vasculitis, cutaneous flushing, exfoliative dermatitis, drug exanthem, contact dermatitis

Nitroprusside

exanthem, purpura, hyperhidrosis

Nizatidine

exanthem, pruritus, hyperhidrosis, purpura, urticaria, exfoliative dermatitis

Norfloxacin

exanthem, erythema, TEN, erythema multiforme major (Stevens-Johnson syndrome), erythema multiforme minor, exfoliative dermatitis, pruritus, photosensitivity, pustular eruption

Nortriptyline

exanthem, pruritus, urticaria, angioedema, black hairy tongue, purpura, petechiae, itching, alopecia, photosensitivity, hyperhidrosis, flushing

Nystatin

fixed drug eruption, erythema multiforme major (Stevens-Johnson syndrome), perioral dermatitis, pruritus

Ofloxacin

diaphoresis, vasculitis, photosensitivity, angioedema, erythema, pruritus, exanthem, anaphylaxis, urticaria

Omeprazole

exanthem, lichen spinulosus

Oral contraceptive agents (combination and sequential)

exanthem, pruritus, urticaria, angioedema, fixed drug eruption, dermatitis, erythema multiforme minor, vesicular or bullous eruption, vasculitis, erythema nodosum, lupus erythematosus, oral mucous membrane lesions, lichenoid eruption, alopecia, hypertrichosis, hirsutism, acneiform eruption, photosensitivity, acanthosis nigricans, induction of porphyria cutanea tarda, candidiasis, melasma, herpes gestationis, melanoma, purpura, seborrhea, spider angiomas, telangiectasia, varicose veins, onycholysis

Oxacillin

exanthem, pruritus, urticaria, vesicular or bullous eruption, oral mucous membrane lesions

Oxazepam

exanthem, pruritus

Oxymetholone

hirsutism, acne

Oxytetracycline

exanthem, pruritus, urticaria, angioedema, fixed drug eruption, purpura, vasculitis, lupus erythematosus, oral mucous membrane lesions, *photosensitivity,* pseudoporphyria, pustular eruption

Oxytocin

urticaria, exanthem, angioedema, anaphylactoid reaction

Pancuronium

diffuse erythema

Papaverine

exanthem, intense flushing of face, hyperhidrosis

Paraben

pruritus, dermatitis, contact dermatitis

Paramethadione

exanthem, pruritus, fixed drug eruption, erythema multiforme minor, purpura, oral mucous membrane lesions, acneiform eruption, exfoliative dermatitis, alopecia

Penicillamine

exanthem, pruritus, urticaria, dermatitis, *erythema multiforme minor,* vesicular or bullous eruption, pemphigus, pemphigoid-like eruption, TEN, purpura, vasculitis, erythema nodosum, lupus erythematosus, oral or genital ulcers, lichenoid eruption, alopecia, hirsutism, exfoliative dermatitis, anetoderma, aphthous stomatitis, yellow nail syndrome, seborrheic dermatitis-like exanthem, contact dermatitis, cutis laxa, dermatomyositis, elastosis perferans serpiginosa, epidermal inclusion cysts, morphea-like eruption, pseudoxanthoma elasticum-like eruption, psoriasiform eruption, systemic sclerosis, hypertrichosis, flushing, atrophic wrinkled skin, easy bruising, milia

Penicillins

exanthem, pruritus, urticaria, angioedema, fixed drug eruption, dermatitis, *erythema multiforme minor,* erythema multiforme major (Stevens-Johnson syndrome), *vesicular or bullous eruption,* TEN, purpura, vasculitis, erythema nodosum, *lupus erythematosus, oral mucous membrane lesions,* lichenoid eruption, acneiform eruption, pemphigus, bullous pemphigoid, pityriasis rosea-like eruption, cutis laxa, hyperhidrosis, exfoliative dermatitis, *photosensitivity, alopecia,* contact dermatitis, pustular psoriasis, erythema annulare centrifugum-like eruption, anaphylaxis, polyarteritis nodosa-like syndrome; at injection site: atrophy, necrosis, wheals

Pentaerythritol tetranitrate

exanthem, fixed drug eruption, dermatitis, cutaneous vasodilation with flushing, exacerbation of rosacea

Pentagastrin

exanthem, pruritus, angioedema, tingling feeling, hyperhidrosis, burning

Pentamidine (IV)

exanthem, erythroderma, sterile abscess at injection site, erythema multiforme major (Stevens-Johnson syndrome), gingivitis, oral ulcer, vasculitis, pruritus, urticaria. Morbilliform exanthem, erythema, xerosis, desquamation, blepharitis, urticaria have also occurred with use of inhaled aerosolized pentamidine.

Pentazocine

exanthem, pruritus, urticaria, angioedema, TEN, diaphoresis, flushing, dermatitis, hyperhidrosis; at injection site: sclerosis with deep ulceration, nodules, hyperpigmentation, granulomas

Pentobarbital

fixed drug eruption, exanthem, angioedema, exfoliative dermatitis, pemphigus, isolated blisters or bullous eruption, erythema multiforme minor, urticaria

Pentoxifylline

exanthem, pruritus, urticaria, angioedema, brittle fingernails

Perphenazine

exanthem, urticaria, angioedema, purpura, lupus erythematosus, dermatitis, exfoliative dermatitis, pruritus, contact dermatitis, hyperpigmentation, photosensitivity

Phenazopyridine

exanthem, yellow-orange or blue-gray change in skin color

Phenelzine

exanthem, *pruritus,* angioedema, purpura, lupus erythematosus, hyperhidrosis, *photosensitivity, glossitis,* xerostomia

Phenobarbital

exanthem, pruritus, urticaria, angioedema, fixed drug eruption, erythema multiforme minor, erythema multiforme major (Stevens-Johnson syndrome), vesicular or bullous eruption, TEN, purpura, vasculitis, erythema nodosum, oral mucous membrane lesions, acneiform eruption, hypohidrosis, flushing, lupus erythematosus, pellagra, photosensitivity, induction of porphyria cutanea tarda, pemphigus, exfoliative dermatitis, alopecia

Phenolphthalein

exanthem, pruritus, *urticaria,* angioedema, *fixed drug eruption,* dermatitis, erythema multiforme minor, vesicular or bullous eruption, TEN, purpura, vasculitis, lupus erythematosus, oral mucous membrane lesions, alopecia, exfoliative dermatitis, changes of skin color—dark gray macules

Phenoxybenzamine

exanthem, pruritus, urticaria, xerostomia

Phensuximide

exanthem, pruritus, erythema multiforme minor, erythema multiforme major (Stevens-Johnson syndrome), purpura, alopecia

Phenytoin (diphenylhydantoin)

exanthem, pruritus, urticaria, angioedema, fixed drug eruption, dermatitis, erythema multiforme minor, erythema multiforme major (Stevens-Johnson syndrome), vesicular or bullous eruption, TEN, purpura, vasculitis, lupus erythematosus, *oral mucous membrane lesions,* lichenoid eruption, *melasma-like hypermelanosis,* hypopigmentation, coarsening of facial features, exfoliative dermatitis, acneiform eruption, pseudolymphoma/lymphoma, *hypertrichosis,* hirsutism, spotty pigmentation, nail malformations, photosensitivity, pellagra-like eruption, alopecia, *gingival hyperplasia,* heel pad thickening, erythroderma, toxic erythema

Pimozide

exanthem, angioedema, xerostomia, hyperhidrosis

Pindolol

dermatitis, vasculitis, lupus erythematosus, lichenoid eruption, pruritus, *exanthem,* hyperhidrosis, psoriasiform eruption

Piroxicam

exanthem, pruritus, acneiform eruption, alopecia, hyperhidrosis, vesiculobullous/photodistributed eruption, burning, stinging, urticaria, photosensitivity (pseudoporphyria), erythema, bruising, desquamation, exfoliative dermatitis, erythema multiforme minor, erythema multiforme major (Stevens-Johnson syndrome), TEN, vasculitis, isolated blisters or bullous eruption, fixed drug eruption, angioedema, Henoch-Schoenlein purpura, erythema annulare centrifugum, pemphigus

Polymyxin B

exanthem, pruritus, urticaria

Prazosin

exanthem, pruritus, urticaria, lupus erythematosus, erythema multiforme minor, alopecia, lichen planus, *xerostomia,* hyperhidrosis, lichenoid eruption, erythema nodosum, anaphylaxis

Prednisolone (see also prednisone)
exanthem, urticaria, fixed drug eruption, ecchymoses, necrosis following injection, angioedema

Prednisone
exanthem, urticaria, angioedema, dermatitis, vesicular or bullous eruption, TEN, *purpura,* acneiform eruption, impaired wound healing, fragile skin, petechiae, *ecchymoses,* facial erythema, hyperhidrosis, porokeratosis (DSAP), *acne/acneiform eruption, hirsutism, striae,* poststeroidal panniculitis, spotty hyperpigmentation, cutaneous infections (children)

Primaquine phosphate
exanthem, pruritus, urticaria, angioedema

Primodone
exanthem, angioedema, erythema multiforme minor, TEN, lupus erythematosus, exfoliative dermatitis

Probenecid
exanthem, pruritus, urticaria, oral mucous membrane lesions, dermatitis, alopecia, xerostomia

Probucol
exanthem, pruritus, angioedema, purpura, ecchymoses, petechiae, hyperhidrosis, fetid sweat

Procainamide
exanthem, pruritus, *urticaria,* angioedema, purpura, vasculitis, *lupus erythematosus,* flushing, eczematous eruption

Procaine
exanthem, pruritus, urticaria, angioedema, dermatitis, erythema multiforme minor, purpura, TEN, photosensitivity, contact dermatitis, wheals at injection site

Procaine penicillin
exanthem, *urticaria,* TEN, bullous eruption. Also see penicillins (p. 146)

Procarbazine
exanthem, pruritus, *urticaria,* angioedema, dermatitis, TEN, purpura, *oral mucous membrane lesions,* herpes simplex, dermatitis, alopecia, hyperpigmentation, photosensitivity, flushing "Antabuse-like" effect

Prochlorperazine
exanthem, urticaria, angioedema, purpura, lupus erythematosus, oral mucous membrane lesions, hypermelanosis, pruritus, eczema, fixed drug eruption, photosensitivity

Progesterone derivatives

exanthem, pruritus, urticaria, angioedema, dermatitis, erythema multiforme minor, vesicular or bullous eruption, oral mucous membrane lesions, melasma, acneiform eruption, alopecia, hirsutism

Promazine

exanthem, urticaria, angioedema, photosensitivity

Promethazine

exanthem, pruritus, urticaria, dermatitis, vesicular or bullous eruption, TEN, purpura, lupus erythematosus, xerostomia, photosensitivity, contact dermatitis, fixed drug eruption

Propoxyphene

exanthem, urticaria

Propranolol

exanthem, pruritus, urticaria, dermatitis, purpura, lichenoid eruption, hypermelanosis of tongue, alopecia, acneiform eruption, psoriasiform exanthem, exacerbation of psoriasis, pemphigus, Raynaud's phenomenon, erythema multiforme minor, lupus erythematosus, Peyrone's disease, TEN

Propylthiouracil

exanthem, pruritus, urticaria, *angioedema,* vasculitis, *lupus erythematosus,* lichenoid eruption, hypermelanosis, alopecia, purpura, agranulocytosis, photosensitivity, fixed drug eruption, bleaching of hair color

Protamine sulfate

flushing, exanthem, urticaria

Protamine-Zinc-Insulin

exanthem, pruritus, urticaria, angioedema, vesicular or bullous eruption, purpura, nodules at injection site

Protriptyline

exanthem, pruritus, urticaria, *dermatitis,* purpura, petechiae, edema, alopecia, photosensitivity

Pyrazinamide

exanthem, urticaria, purpura, reddish brown changes in skin color, photosensitivity, alopecia, flushing, exacerbation of porphyria cutanea tarda

Pyrimethamine

exanthem, vesicular or bullous eruption, purpura, photosensitivity, oral mucous membrane lesions, dermatitis, hypermelanosis, TEN, lichenoid eruption, pustular eruption

Quinacrine

exanthem, lichenoid eruption, exfoliative dermatitis, *pruritus,* aggravated psoriasis, alopecia, *dermatitis,* isolated blisters or bullous eruption, *urticaria,* fixed drug eruption, erythema annulare centrifugum, porphyria cutanea tarda, exacerbation of psoriasis, erythema multiforme minor, pigmentary changes of nails, skin, palate including *yellowish discoloration of skin*

Quinestrol

urticaria, angioedema, melasma, erythema multiforme minor, erythema nodosum, hemorrhagic eruption, alopecia, hirsutism

Quinethazone

purpura, photosensitivity, exanthem, urticaria, vasculitis, isolated blisters or bullous eruption

Quinidine

exanthem, pruritus, urticaria angioedema, fixed drug eruption, dermatitis, erythema multiforme minor, vesicular or bullous eruption, TEN, *purpura,* vasculitis, photosensitivity, lupus erythematosus, oral mucous membrane lesions, anaphylaxis, lichenoid photosensitive eruption, alopecia, blue-gray discoloration of nails, pretibial skin and hard palate; exfoliative dermatitis, exacerbation of psoriasis, acneiform eruption, thrombocytopenic purpura

Quinine

exanthem, pruritus, *urticaria, angioedema,* fixed drug eruption, dermatitis, erythema multiforme minor, erythema multiforme major (Stevens-Johnson syndrome), vesicular or bullous eruption, TEN, purpura, vasculitis, photosensitivity, lupus erythematosus, oral mucous membrane lesions, anaphylaxis, lichenoid eruption in photodistributed areas, acneiform eruption, flushing, hyperhidrosis, livedo reticularis-like photosensitive eruption, alopecia

Ranitidine

exanthem, erythema multiforme minor, alopecia, urticaria, edema, pruritus, vasculitis, angioedema, pustular eruption, dermatitis

Reserpine

exanthem, urticaria, angioedema, fixed drug eruption, purpura, lupus erythematosus, alopecia, pruritus, flushing, hyperhidrosis, photosensitivity, xerostomia

Ribavirin

exanthem, fixed eruption, erythema multiforme minor

Rifampin

exanthem, pruritus, urticaria, angioedema, erythema multiforme minor, vesicular or bullous eruption, purpura, lupus erythematosus, oral mucous membrane lesions, sore mouth, sore tongue, orange-red discoloration of skin, exudative conjunctivitis, pemphigus, *flushing,* bullous pemphigoid-like reaction, TEN, exfoliative dermatitis, porphyria cutanea tarda, vasculitis, anaphylaxis, *acne in men*

Ritodrine
dermatitis, erythema, hyperhidrosis

Salicylamide
vesicular or bullous eruption, TEN

Salsalate
exanthem, angioedema, urticaria, hyperhidrosis

Secobarbital
exanthem, angioedema, exfoliative dermatitis

Secretin
urticaria

Silver
oral mucous membrane lesions, changes in skin color (argyria), skin necrosis, erythema multiforme minor, photosensitivity

Simvastatin
angioedema, lupus erythematosus-like syndrome, purpura, urticaria, photosensitivity, flushing, TEN, erythema multiforme minor, alopecia

Somatostatin
purpura

Spectinomycin
exanthem, pruritus, urticaria, oral mucous membrane lesions, induration at injection site

Spironolactone
exanthem, urticaria, lichenoid eruption, alopecia, purpura, Raynaud's phenomenon, melasma-like pigmentation, pruritus, xerosis, erythema annulare centrifugum, vasculitis

Stanazolol
edema, hirsutism, acne, alopecia

Streptokinase
exanthem, urticaria, dermatitis, vasculitis, oral mucous membrane lesions, pruritus, flushing, leukocytoclastic vasculitis, angioedema, serum sickness, *phlebitis* at injection site

Streptomycin

exanthem, pruritus, urticaria, angioedema, fixed drug eruption, dermatitis, erythema multiforme minor, erythema multiforme major (Stevens-Johnson syndrome), vesicular or bullous eruption, TEN, purpura, vasculitis, erythema nodosum, lupus erythematosus, oral mucous membrane lesions, lichenoid eruption, hypertrichosis, acneiform eruption, exfoliative dermatitis, photosensitivity, induration at injection site

Streptozocin

exanthem, pruritus, oral mucous membrane lesions, TEN

Succinylcholine

urticaria, exanthem

Sucralfate

pruritus, exanthem

Sulfadoxine

exanthem, urticaria, dermatitis, erythema multiforme minor, vesicular or bullous eruption, TEN, photosensitivity, lupus erythematosus, pruritus, exfoliative dermatitis

Sulfamethizole

exanthem, pruritus, urticaria, erythema multiforme minor, TEN

Sulfamethoxazole

exanthem, pruritus, urticaria, angioedema, fixed drug eruption, erythema multiforme minor, vesicular or bullous eruption, purpura, erythema nodosum, TEN, exfoliative dermatitis, periorbital edema, pustular eruption, lupus erythematosus

Sulfamethoxypyridazine

exanthem, pruritus, *urticaria,* erythema multiforme minor, erythema multiforme major (Stevens-Johnson syndrome), fixed drug eruption, isolated blisters or bullous eruption, erythema nodosum, TEN, purpura, photosensitivity, lupus erythematosus

Sulfasalazine

exanthem, dermatitis, bluish or yellowish skin discoloration, erythema multiforme minor, erythema multiforme major (Stevens-Johnson syndrome), vesicular or bullous eruption, TEN, vasculitis, lupus erythematosus, urticaria, pruritus, *psoriasiform* eruption, oral ulcers, exfoliative dermatitis, photosensitivity, Raynaud's phenomenon, alopecia

Sulfathiazole

pruritus, urticaria, fixed drug eruption, vesicular or bullous eruption, TEN, erythema nodosum, oral mucous membrane lesions, photosensitivity, lupus erythematosus

Sulfinpyrazone
exanthem

Sulfisoxazole
photosensitivity, fixed drug eruption, *exanthem,* pruritus, urticaria, angioedema, erythema multiforme minor, vesicular or bullous eruption, TEN, purpura, vasculitis, lupus erythematosus, oral mucous membrane lesions, edema, porphyria cutanea tarda, exfoliative dermatitis

Sulindac
exanthem, pruritus, angioedema, oral mucous membrane lesions, stomatitis, alopecia, photosensitivity, purpura, hyperhidrosis, exfoliative erythroderma, urticaria, petechiae, lichenoid eruption, fixed drug eruption, TEN, erythema multiforme major (Stevens-Johnson syndrome), serum sickness, facial/oral erythema, pernio-like reaction, vasculitis

Suramin sodium
exanthem, pruritus, urticaria, angioedema, keratoacanthoma, actinic porokeratosis, *oral mucous membrane lesions* in patients with AIDS

Tamoxifen
exanthem, purpura, *alopecia, flushing,* edema, xerostomia, vasculitis, xerosis

Tartrazine
urticaria, vasculitis

Taxol
exanthem, pruritus, *urticaria,* angioedema, *alopecia,* flushing, *oral mucous membrane lesions*

Terbutaline
hyperhidrosis, exanthem, flushing, vasculitis

Testosterone
exanthem, urticaria, acneiform eruption, hirsutism, lupus erythematosus, exacerbation of porphyria cutanea tarda, alopecia

Tetracycline
exanthem, pruritus, urticaria, angioedema, fixed drug eruption, dermatitis, erythema multiforme minor, erythema multiforme major (Stevens-Johnson syndrome), vesicular or bullous eruption, purpura, vasculitis, lupus erythematosus, oral mucous membrane lesions, lichenoid eruption, acneiform eruption, phototoxic reaction, photo-onycholysis, blue-gray pigmentation, hyperhidrosis, TEN, exfoliative dermatitis, postacne osteoma cutis, pseudoporphyria, psoriasis induction or exacerbation

Thallium
oral mucous membrane lesions, alopecia

Theophylline

exanthem, dermatitis, erythema multiforme major (Stevens-Johnson syndrome)

Thiabendazole

exanthem, pruritus, *urticaria,* angioedema, dermatitis, erythema multiforme minor, erythema multiforme major (Stevens-Johnson syndrome), TEN, oral mucous membrane lesions, spotty hypermelanosis, facial flush, fixed drug eruption

Thiacetazone

exanthem, pruritus, urticaria, angioedema, desquamation, bullae, TEN, erythema multiforme major (Stevens-Johnson syndrome), alopecia

Thiethylperazine

erythema, exfoliative dermatitis, contact dermatitis

Thioguanine

oral mucous membrane lesions, exanthem, photosensitivity, alopecia

Thiopental

exanthem, urticaria, angioedema, erythema multiforme minor, erythema multiforme major (Stevens-Johnson syndrome), vesicular or bullous eruption, purpura, fixed drug eruption, anaphylaxis

Thioridazine

exanthem, angioedema, dermatitis, vasculitis, lupus erythematosus, slate gray skin color, hirsutism, urticarial eruption, erythema, exfoliative dermatitis, photosensitivity

Thiotepa

exanthem, pruritus, *urticaria,* angioedema, purpura, oral mucous membrane lesions, depigmentation, alopecia, hyperpigmentation under occluded skin, redness and burning, bullae, mild erythema

Thiothixene

exanthem, pruritus, urticaria, *xerostomia,* exfoliative dermatitis, photosensitivity

Ticlopidine

exanthem, purpura, urticaria, vasculitis, lupus erythematosus (positive ANA), serum sickness

Tiopronin

exanthem, pruritus, vesicular or bullous eruption, vasculitis, lichenoid eruption, erythema, urticaria, pemphigus, lupus erythematosus, stomatitis, *photosensitivity,* alopecia

Tobramycin
exanthem, pruritus, exfoliative dermatitis

Tolazamide
exanthem, pruritus, dermatitis, erythema, lichenoid eruption, lupus erythematosus, urticaria

Tolazoline
flushing, exanthem

Tolbutamide
exanthem, pruritus, urticaria, fixed drug eruption, dermatitis, erythema multiforme minor, vesicular or bullous eruption, TEN, purpura, erythema nodosum, lupus erythematosus, lichenoid eruption, photosensitivity, induction of porphyria cutanea tarda

Tolmetin
exanthem, pruritus, urticaria, irritation, anaphylactoid reaction, purpura, erythema multiforme minor, TEN, anaphylaxis

Tranylcypromine
exanthem, pruritus, dermatitis, edema, induction of porphyria cutanea tarda

Triamcinolone
hirsutism, acneiform eruption, folliculitis, purpura, *ecchymoses,* hypertrichosis, hypopigmentation, skin atrophy, *striae,* miliaria, petechiae, erythema, lipoatrophy, urticaria

Triamterene
exanthem, urticaria, purpura, photosensitivity, subacute cutaneous lupus erythematosus (reported in combination with hydrochlorothiazide therapy)

Trihexyphenidyl
exanthem, xerostomia

Trimethadione
exanthem, pruritus, urticaria, fixed drug eruption, erythema multiforme minor, vesicular or bullous eruption, purpura, lupus erythematosus, oral mucous membrane lesions, alopecia, acneiform eruption or exacerbation of acne, exfoliative dermatitis, photosensitivity

Trimethoprim
exanthem, urticaria, purpura, exanthem, pruritus, erythema nodosum, photosensitivity, anaphylaxis, TEN, erythema multiforme minor, erythema multiforme major (Stevens-Johnson syndrome), fixed drug eruption

Trimethoprim + Sulfamethoxazole

exanthem, pruritus, urticaria, dermatitis, erythema multiforme minor, erythema multiforme major (Stevens-Johnson syndrome), vesicular or bullous eruption, TEN, vasculitis, *oral mucous membrane lesions including glossitis and erosions,* purpura, photosensitivity, pustular reaction, lupus erythematosus, pustular toxic erythema, exfoliative dermatitis, *angioedema,* Henoch-Schoenlein purpura, serum sickness, conjunctival and scleral injection, periarteritis nodosa-like syndrome, fixed drug eruption

Tripelennamine

exanthem, urticaria, angioedema, fixed drug eruption, dermatitis, purpura, photosensitivity, lichenoid eruption, pityriasis rosea-like eruption

Triprolidine

exanthem, angioedema, lichenoid eruption, urticaria, photosensitivity, xerostomia, dryness of nose and throat

Tumor Necrosis Factor

local reaction at injection site, skin necrosis or ulceration

Urokinase

exanthem

Vaccine: BCG

exanthem, urticaria, dermatitis, erythema multiforme minor, vesicular or bullous eruption, TEN, purpura, vasculitis, erythema nodosum, lupus erythematosus, disseminated tuberculosis, porokeratosis at vaccination site

Vaccine: Cholera

exanthem, pruritus, urticaria, dermatitis, vesicular or bullous eruption, lichenoid eruption; at injection site: erythema, induration, pain and tenderness

Vaccine: Diphtheria antitoxin

TEN

Vaccine DTP: Diphtheria-Pertussis-Tetanus Toxoid

exanthem, urticaria, angioedema, erythema nodosum, erythema multiforme minor, erythema multiforme major (Stevens-Johnson syndrome), dermatitis, TEN, purpura; at injection site: erythema, swelling, induration, pain, sterile abscess or subcutaneous atrophy

Vaccine: Hepatitis B

urticaria, exanthem

Vaccine: Influenza

urticaria, angioedema, purpura, vasculitis; at injection site: hives, lupus erythematosus, slight tenderness, redness, induration

Vaccine: Measles

exanthem, urticaria, erythema multiforme minor, erythema multiforme major (Stevens-Johnson syndrome), TEN, purpura, exfoliative dermatitis; at injection site: short duration burning/stinging

Vaccine: Mumps/Parotitis

urticaria, erythema multiforme minor; at injection site: short duration burning/stinging

Vaccine: Poliomyelitis (Sabin)

urticaria, angioedema, dermatitis

Vaccine: Poliomyelitis (Salk)

exanthem, urticaria, angioedema, dermatitis, erythema multiforme minor, TEN, purpura, vasculitis, erythema nodosum

Vaccine: Rabies

exanthem, pruritus, urticaria, angioedema, purpura, vasculitis

Vaccine: Rubella (German Measles)

exanthem, vasculitis

Vaccine: Tetanus antitoxin

urticaria, TEN, erythema nodosum, lupus erythematosus

Vaccine: Tularemia

dermatitis, vesicular or bullous eruption

Vaccine: Typhus/Paratyphus

exanthem, urticaria, angioedema, fixed drug eruption, dermatitis, purpura, lupus erythematosus

Valproic acid

exanthem, purpura, *transient alopecia,* photosensitivity, erythema multiforme minor, hypertrichosis, pruritus, curling of hair, scleroderma-like/morphea-like changes, vasculitis

Vancomycin

exanthem, pruritus, *urticaria,* angioedema, exfoliative dermatitis, erythema multiforme major (Stevens-Johnson syndrome), flushing, linear IgA bullous dermatosis, vasculitis, bullous eruption, "Red Man syndrome," TEN, thrombophlebitis at injection site

Vasopressin

urticaria, angioedema, hyperhidrosis; at injection site: cutaneous gangrene/necrosis

Verapamil

exanthem, pruritus, angioedema, photosensitivity, purpura, vasculitis, xerostomia, arthralgia and exanthem, alopecia, hyperkeratosis, hyperhidrosis, urticaria, erythema multiforme minor, erythema multiforme major (Stevens-Johnson syndrome), psoriasiform exanthem, *flushing*, lichenoid eruption

Vidarabine

exanthem, pruritus, purpura

Vinblastine

dermatitis, vesicular or bullous eruption, *oral mucous membrane lesions*, acneiform eruption, *alopecia*, skin vesiculation, Raynaud's phenomenon, photosensitivity, isolated blisters or bullous eruption; intralesional injection results in pain, redness, swelling with necrosis of injected lesions at 36-48 hrs

Vincristine

exanthem, pruritus, *oral mucous membrane lesions*, edema, *alopecia;* pain, redness, swelling at injection site

Vitamin A (Retinol)

exanthem, pruritus, dermatitis, erythema multiforme minor, purpura, photosensitivity, oral mucous membrane lesions, alopecia, acneiform eruption

Vitamin B Complex

pruritus, urticaria, dermatitis

Vitamin B$_1$ (Thiamine)

exanthem, pruritus, urticaria, angioedema, dermatitis, purpura

Vitamin B$_2$ (Riboflavin)

acneiform eruption

Vitamin B$_3$ (Niacin) - see nicotinic acid

Vitamin B$_6$ (Pyridoxine)

acneiform eruption, vasculitis

Vitamin B$_{12}$ (Cyanocobalamine)

pruritus, urticaria, angioedema, dermatitis, vesicular or bullous eruption, acneiform eruption, flushing, induction of porphyria cutanea tarda

Vitamin C (Ascorbic acid)

exanthem, pruritus, urticaria, angioedema

Vitamin D$_2$ (Calciferol)

exanthem, pruritus, urticaria, dermatitis, erythema nodosum, acneiform eruption

Vitamin E (Tocoferol)

urticaria, dermatitis

Vitamin K₁ (Phytonadione)

exanthem, urticaria, purpura, vasculitis hyperhidrosis; at injection site: pain/swelling, erythematous plaques that may become sclerodermatous

Vitamin K₃ (Menadione)

urticaria, vasculitis, exanthem

VP16 - see etoposide

Warfarin

exanthem, pruritus, urticaria, dermatitis, vesicular or bullous eruption, purpura, oral mucous membrane lesions, alopecia, cutaneous necrosis, acral purple erythema that may be reticulated

Zidovudine

exanthem, acne or acneiform eruption, oral mucous membrane lesions including oral ulcers, *pruritus,* urticaria, *brown, blackish or bluish nail discoloration, diffuse or striate,* bluish lunulae, vasculitis, bullous lesions, hyperpigmentation of skin and mucous membranes, porphyria cutanea tarda, eyelash hypertrichosis, erythema multiforme major (Stevens-Johnson syndrome), oral ulcers